Targeting Intelligible Speech

Itis Mennie

TARGETING INTELLIGIBLE SPEECH

A Phonological Approach to Remediation

by
Barbara Williams Hodson
San Diego State University

and
Elaine Pagel Paden
University of Illinois, Urbana-Champaign

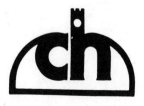

College-Hill Press
San Diego, California

College-Hill Press, Inc.
4284 41st Street
San Diego, CA 92105

Library of Congress Cataloging in Publication Data

Hodson, Barbara Williams.
   Targeting Intelligible Speech.

   Bibliography: p.
   Includes index.
   1. Speech therapy for children. 2. Phonetics.
I. Paden, Elaine Pagel. II. Title.
RJ496.S7H55   1982   618. 92′85506   82-19863

ISBN   0-933014-81-3

Printed in the United States of America

TABLE OF CONTENTS

TABLES

EXERCISES

FOREWORD

Since I took my first course in articulation disorders as an undergraduate, almost twenty years ago, much has happened in this field. In fact, in some programs, a course entitled something like "Disorders of Articulation" is no longer a part of the curriculum; instead, we find a course with a title like "Phonological Disorders." Phonology has emerged as a vital and significant part of academic training in speech and language disorders and as a powerful tool in the assessment and management of these disorders. This emergence has been marked by several recent books on phonology that have been written for the speech-language pathologist.

Barbara Hodson and Elaine Paden's *Targeting Intelligible Speech* is a major step in describing, explaining, and justifying the phonological approach. Most of the ideas in this new book were born in the clinical experiences of the authors. This invaluable clinical experience, combined with Hodson and Paden's awareness of a complex and rapidly growing literature on phonological analysis and phonological development, gives their book freshness, depth, and relevance. As readers, we benefit not only from the authors' knowledge tested by experience in the clinical proving ground, but also from their sensitivity to the unanswered questions, to lacunae, and to controversy. There is much in this book that is practical; and there is also a cautious respect for what we do not yet know. To achieve this combination is a major challenge in education. On the one hand, we must give our students competence and confidence in what they can do with today's knowledge; on the other hand, we must encourage them to think independently, to hold fast that which meets the test of application, and to seek continually for a better way. I think that *Targeting Intelligible Speech*, is written in this vein.

Even twenty years ago, when the traditional phonemic approach was taught to my generation of speech-language pathologists, there was a realization that *patterns of error* held the key to efficient and effective management. Hodson and Paden show us that phonological analysis gives us a greater sophistication in identifying and manipulating deficient patterns of speech. The authors work systematically through major issues in the phonological approach, defining the what, the how, and the why of phonological analysis. The bulk of this book is devoted to the biggest challenge, that of explaining how speech-language pathologists can use phonological analysis to design and evaluate an intervention procedure. The authors describe a remediation method based on "cycle programming." Contrary to many remediation programs that rely on continued training of individual targets until proficiency is established, cycle programming focuses on a particular target for a relatively short time, then moves on to a new target, and so on, until sequential targeting of several patterns has been accomplished. Subsequent cycles are essentially review cycles and may be repeated until satisfactory performance is achieved for each target. This remediation program is carefully documented and is illustrated with six case studies. Along the way, Hodson and Paden give many useful hints and facts pertaining to phonological analysis and to phonological development in children. The book is rich in information, clear in presentation, and logical in structure.

Targeting Intelligible Speech draws together many threads to show how a phonological approach to the remediation of deficient patterns in children's speech can lead to a systematic, individualized program of intervention. The book is an asset to the field and a welcome addition to the bookshelf of every phonologist or speech-language pathologist.

Ray D. Kent

PREFACE

This book has been written in response to requests from speech-language pathologists who work with children with severe articulation disorders. It is designed for the practicing clinician and also for the student in training. The goal is to share information we have accumulated while working with over 100 highly unintelligible children, which has helped us to expedite intelligibility gains. The children we are referring to are those whose connected speech utterances are estimated to be less than 15% intelligible by adult listeners.

Our profession has very effectively served children with mild to moderate speech disorders. However, our record as a whole with children who have severe to profound articulation deficiencies is generally less a source of pride. Extraordinary amounts of time have been expended, and considerable frustration seems to have been experienced by clinicians, clients, families, and teachers during the long terms of programming which elapsed before these children could function satisfactorily in school and society.

We also observed that even as phonological research was expanding, most remediation programs for unintelligible children were still targeting phoneme *segments* rather than phonological *systems*. Typically, a phoneme was chosen for a reason such as "age of singleton phoneme acquisition norms," "visibility," "inconsistent productions," etc., and then the phoneme was "perfected," first in the initial position, next in final position, then in medial position, and, sometimes, in consonant clusters. Eventually, the children learned each singleton phoneme, but the process could best be described as laborious. In addition, it has been observed that at the end of their remediation programs these children often produced single words satisfactorily, but their systems frequently "broke down" in conversational utterances.

In the mid-1970s we decided to initiate a "Phonology Program," which accepted only highly unintelligible children. The "state of the art" at that time led us at first to analyze and teach distinctive features and phonological rules. We soon found that while features and rules made contributions, they were not sufficiently encompassing for the needs of highly unintelligible children. We then looked at the concept of "natural processes," but found that unintelligible children's speech samples often contained complex patterns which could not be explained adequately as simplifications of adult speech. We therefore developed an analytical system which allowed us to specify uncommon deficient patterns as well as the more common ones. We found that once we could account for the child's whole phonological system, we could ascertain which patterns most needed to be targeted. We found it unnecessary to target every pattern, and we did not attempt to perfect every phoneme. Rather, we decided which patterns were critical and set out to remediate them in a systematic manner.

The Phonology Program described in this book evolved over a period of six years. Clinical research hypotheses were formulated, tested, accepted, or rejected; conclusions were drawn or hypotheses were re-formulated and tested as required by the obtained results. We recognize the value of controlled studies, but we were unwilling to withhold phonological programming from any unintelligible client who requested service, even for the purpose of having matched controls. We felt that time was of the essence for these unintelligible clients and that they deserved the best remediation service currently available in our clinic.

Even though speech disorders have been around for a long time and articulation intervention has undergone many changes, the phonological approach to remediation is relatively new. In fact, we consider it to be in its embryonic stage of development. What we are sharing in this book is certainly not the final word. We anticipate the continued refinement of this program, and we especially recognize the need to make adaptations for those children with profound intellectual and/or physical involvements. We expect possibly dramatic changes to occur in the next few years, and we invite clinicians in all professional environments to help us continue to grow and to develop improved methods to better serve unintelligible children.

The reader may observe that our children will be referred to as "he" whenever the term "they" is too cumbersome. Since there were more xiii

than twice as many boys as girls in our Phonology Program, and all of the six clients whose case histories are included in this volume are boys, "he" seems to be the appropriate singular pronoun. Following this same reasoning, the speech-language pathologist who works with children is referred to as "she."

We are particularly indebted to several individuals who assisted us in the preparation of this book. Robert K. Simpson, Carla Euliss, JoAnn Higgs, and Elizabeth Miller read the manuscript and provided valuable suggestions. Ilene Siegel and Jean Ommen Gill meticulously checked client data. W.R. Zemlin generously contributed his skill in photography, and the University of Illinois News Bureau provided four of the pictures. Betty Kempton patiently and expertly assisted in the manuscript preparation. Most of all, we wish to thank our students and our clients, who continually provided us with new insights into phonological disorders and their remediation, as well as our families, who provided support and understanding.

INTRODUCTION

Learning to communicate through language involves the acquisition of skills in four areas: Phonology (sound structure); Semantics (vocabulary and word meaning); Grammar (inflection and syntax); and Pragmatics (communicative exchange). Inadequacy in any of these areas results in communication problems to the extent of the severity of the deficiency, but the particular concern of the specialist in articulation disorders is phonology.

Knowledge about phonology has increased rapidly in recent years, particularly in the area of child phonology. As a more explicit understanding of normal phonological acquisition has emerged, it has become possible to identify more clearly the nature of phonological deviancy. This has been set forth with such thoroughness by David Ingram in his classic *Phonological Disability in Children* (1976) that it will not be included here. Although there is undoubtedly much more to be learned as large numbers of children are studied, the speech-language pathologist now has a more pressing immediate concern: How can new insights into the nature of phonological deviancy be utilized both in the assessment and in the remediation of disordered speech?

A number of publications are available which outline specific methods for phonological assessment. These differ in the method of collecting speech samples for analysis and in analysis procedures. To secure a speech sample, Compton and Hutton (*The Compton-Hutton Phonological Assessment*, 1978) and Weiner (*Phonological Process Analysis*, 1979) employ sets of pictures to elicit specific word responses. Hodson (*The Assessment of Phonological Processes*, 1980) uses three-dimensional objects which are to be named spontaneously. Shriberg and Kwiatkowski (*Natural Process Analysis*, 1980) prefer a connected speech sample obtained in a play situation. Ingram (*Procedures for the Phonological Analysis of Children's*

Language, 1981) indicates that whatever type of transcribed speech is available—a language sample, a day-to-day diary, or even the entire-word responses to a standard articulation test—can be used as the corpus to be analyzed.

As an analysis procedure, Compton and Hutton (1978) prefer to describe the child's system by means of phonemically stated phonological rules (e.g., $\left[\begin{smallmatrix} r \\ \end{smallmatrix}\right] \rightarrow [w] \, / \, \#C \_\_$).

The other published procedures, all of which recommend identifying the phonological processes the child is using, vary somewhat in focus. Shriberg and Kwiatkowski (1980) essentially limit their analysis to eight "natural processes." Weiner (1978) has a longer list of 16 processes for which he provides specific tests. Both of these manuals encourage the examiner to be alert for other patterns which may be occurring, but they do not give many suggestions for what these might be. Hodson (1980) lists over 40 phonological processes which may be designated. Many of these are sub-categories of common general processes. Ingram (1981) recommends a summary of all of the substitutions or omissions which a child has used for each consonant, followed by an identification of each of the processes these represent. He outlines eight basic types of processes, some of which have sub-categories, but describes 19 others which can be identified.

Suggestions for remediation procedures based on phonological principles have only recently begun to appear in the literature. So far, these have consisted primarily of specific techniques for perception and production training (e.g., Blache & Parsons, 1980; Weiner & Bankson, 1978; Weiner, 1981), descriptions of structured programs suggested for feature training (e.g., McReynolds & Bennett, 1972; Costello & Onstine, 1976; Ruder & Bunce, 1981), or single case studies of individual children reporting procedures which were followed with varying results (e.g., Dunn & Barron, 1982). However, the clinician who seeks advice on how to set up a comprehensive, efficient, individualized program for any child with highly unintelligible speech finds very little guidance in the literature. It is this gap which this volume seeks to fill.

The principles which will be set forth in subsequent chapters have been developed during six years of direct day-to-day experience in the remediation of deviant phonological systems in 125 children, whose age range at the time of our initial contact was three to nine years, many who were judged to be virtually unintelligible in connected speech at referral. During this time, we have experimented with and continually refined both approach and techniques. Our present system is the distillation of this experience. It is based upon an empirical appraisal of the relative extent to which removal of various processes affects the child's intelligibility, and the comparative ease with which the new patterns can be established. Most importantly, the procedure has proved to be effective and expedient. The children involved in this program (the majority were judged to be less than 15% intelligible in spontaneous connected utterances at the time of admission) have been dismissed (that is, their speech had become intelligible) in 18 months or less. How this program has been implemented will be described step-by-step. In addition, exercises are provided to facilitate the reader's understanding. The explanations combined with the exercises are designed to prepare the speech-language pathologist to identify the specific needs of a child with multiple misarticulations, and to design and implement a program to expedite his progress toward intelligible speech. For reference purposes, a Glossary is included.

It should be emphasized that the approach summarized in the following chapters was designed, and proved to be successful for children whose intelligibility was severely impaired. It is neither appropriate nor realistic in cases of mild articulation disorder. For the child who substitutes /f/ for /θ/, has no postvocalic /l/, and/or produces a frontal /s/, traditional phoneme-oriented methods seem to be quite adequate. Furthermore, we believe that the remediation of minimal, essentially intelligible deviations is less urgent, timewise, for a young child, as they are not as damaging to communication needs or school progress.

In the following chapters, the general **phonological approach** to evaluating and remediating deviant articulation will first be described. **Deficient patterns in children's speech** will be identified in Chapter 2 while methods of sampling and analyzing speech for the purpose of observing these patterns will be discussed. An explicit procedure for **identifying remediation priorities** will be proposed in Chapter 3, including both a method of quantification of the overall severity of the child's disorder and a scale for determining the priority of patterns for remediation. Chapter 4 will be devoted to **basic remediation concepts and procedures**. A detailed description of our method of **programming remediation** comprises Chapter 5. This program will be illustrated by **case studies** of six clients in Chapter 6, including delineation of their remediation programs. Their pretest and posttest responses and scores appear in the Appendix. Chapter 7 will suggest ways of **adapting the program to the public school setting**.

Chapter 1

The Phonological Approach

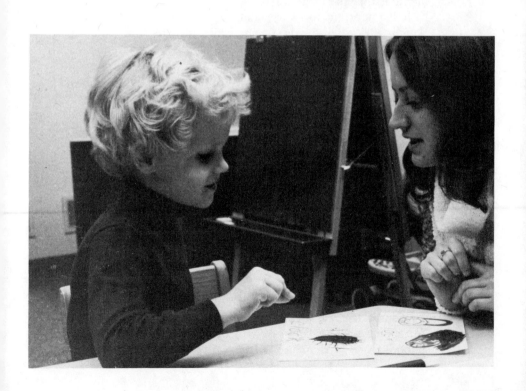

WHAT IS PHONOLOGY?

Phonology deals with the sound structure of language. The structure has two components, a systematic repertoire of meaningful sounds (phonemes) and a finite set of rules defining how these phonemes can be arranged sequentially. Standard adult American English, for example, has 42 phonemes and adheres to such rules as not allowing / ŋ / to begin a word and the requirement for the plural morpheme, -s, to be pronounced / z / when following a voiced phoneme.

We are able to communicate easily with another person who speaks the same language, that is, one who selects sounds from the same repertoire and strings them together in the same arrangements as we do. The more that person's system differs from ours, the more difficult it is for us to understand. Thus, we don't find it hard to converse with someone who speaks another American English dialect, since both of us adhere to the same basic patterns, even though both of us are probably aware of some minor phonetic differences in the "way we talk." Typical British English may at times cause us a few problems, as it includes a number of obvious differences from our own system; while Scottish dialect, which varies even more, may be quite difficult to understand and cockney dialect is close to incomprehensible for most Americans.

It is important to realize that an individual who has any oral language is using sounds systematically, for that is how language is defined. This does not imply, however, that the speaker is overtly conscious of the details of the system he is using. Most adults find it difficult to list, at best, more than four or five of the phonological rules of their own language, even though they follow these rules precisely every time they speak.

By the time most children have acquired a vocabulary of, say, 25 words, they demonstrate an emerging phonological system. The child cannot, of course, immediately learn the entire array of phonemes or the complicated set of sequence patterns of the language he will eventually speak. So he progresses gradually from the mastery of the "simpler" sounds and arrangements to the more complex ones. Just as a child whose vocabulary limitations result in his calling all adult males "Daddy," may say "Ball mine," when only a few of the rules of grammar have been acquired, he will use his few sounds and sound patterns in place of the others he has not yet mastered or simply omit complex sounds and sequences. Child phonologists have observed, however, that a young child makes these substitutions or reductions in generally predictable ways. Thus, even the child's technique for coping with his language inadequacies—that is, developmental phonology—is systematic. In fact, until there is some system in his utterances, he has no language; he is only babbling.

The systematicity of child phonology became more clearly understood when sounds were considered to be made up of groups of distinctive features (Jakobson, Fant, & Halle, 1952; Chomsky & Halle, 1968; Singh, 1976), when various word forms were observed to be the output of the same phonological rule (Smith, 1973; Compton, 1975) and when Stampe's theory of natural processes (1969) suggested common techniques through which children reduce a very complex adult language model to a level with which they can cope. Thus, young children whose systems do not yet include the features continuant and strident often use stop consonants in place of fricatives. (Stampe called this process "Stopping.") If they lack the back feature, children may use alveolar sounds in place of velars ("Fronting"). Until they have expanded the complexity of their syllable structure to include the CCVC form, they will probably produce only CV syllables ("Cluster Reduction" and "Final Consonant Deletion").

People who do not frequently associate with very young children may have difficulty understanding them, not being familiar with the common simplifications children use. Parents and siblings usually have less difficulty as, perhaps without being aware of it, they have identified at least part of the system the child follows, or they know the child's communicative intent. In general, as is the case with dialects, understanding a child is easier when his sound system is similar to our own. Children whose sound structures have many differences from speech which is typical at their stage of development, or who use unusual simplifications or sound combinations, may be essentially unintelligible even to their parents.

THE PHONOLOGY OF DISORDERED SPEECH

Until the mid-1970s, most speech pathologists conceived of disordered speech as the result of phonemic, rather than phonological, differences. They, therefore, simply assessed which phonemes a child had acquired and then attempted to teach, one by one, those that were missing. Although they usually noted when all of the missing sounds were members of a traditional class or classes, such as fricatives or velars, they did not often capitalize upon the systematic nature of the phonemic inadequacies. Furthermore, when viewed as phonemic inadequacies, disordered speech, especially that which was most unintelligible, was described as being "highly inconsistent," even random, in how sounds were used. A child might clearly demonstrate his ability to produce /s/ in some words, yet at other times omit it or substitute one of several other sounds in its place in still other words.

Compton (1970) and Oller (1973) were among the first to demonstrate that children whose speech is highly unintelligible have phonological systems which are just as structured and regular as do children whose speech is developing normally. Each of these children's repertoires of sounds, though typically smaller, represents orderly acquisition and is based upon systematic alterations from the adult model. Each child's rules for syllable structure and for the occurrence of sounds in various positions and in given phonetic environments are basically uniform. In fact, Compton and Oller found that many of the processes found in disordered speech are the same as those which younger normal children use; for example, deletion of final consonants. Therefore, each child's production of any word we have not yet heard him say is predictable, providing his underlying system has been ascertained and he has not already had single-phoneme-oriented intervention which may have contaminated that system. If our prediction is correct, it means that we have been successful in determining the deficient patterns which his sound system is currently following. If our prediction is wrong, however, it does not prove that the child has no system or that he is inconsistent. It simply indicates either that we have not yet adequately analyzed his system, or, perhaps, that at the moment, he is in a stage of transition and therefore is vacillating between patterns. When speech-language pathologists realized that disordered speech, even the most unintelligible, has its own regular structure, the way was opened for a phonological approach to remediation.

THE PHONOLOGICAL APPROACH
TO EVALUATION AND REMEDIATION

The focus of this volume is upon the remediation of articulation of highly unintelligible children. Simply stated, the phonological approach takes advantage of the systematic nature of speech deviations. Rather than focusing on individual sound errors and perfecting phoneme segments, the phonological approach attacks the basic system. Failure to produce /s/, for example, may be the result of different processes in different word situations. It may be omitted at the end of words because the child deletes all postvocalic singleton obstruents (house → /haʊ/), but it may be omitted preceeding another consonant because he omits strident sounds in clusters (stop → /tɑp/). It may be replaced by /t/ in the initial position because the child has not yet acquired the strident or continuant feautres (some → /tʌm/), or by /d/ if he also voices all prevocalic obstruents (some → /dʌm/), or by /k/ if backing or velar assimilation occurs (some → /kʌm/; sock → /kɑk/). Teaching /s/ as an isolated unit, therefore, does not assure its correct use in all of these situations.

On the other hand, remediating a phonological process in a young child's speech can influence all of the sounds that are similarly affected, providing some other process does not intervene. "Acquiring new sound patterns" describes more accurately the way a child learns speech naturally rather than to say he is "learning sounds." Phonology therefore provides a logical approach to training when the child has, for whatever reason, failed to acquire normal speech patterns on his own. It is upon this premise that the procedures described in the next chapters are based.

Chapter 2

Deficient Patterns in Children's Speech

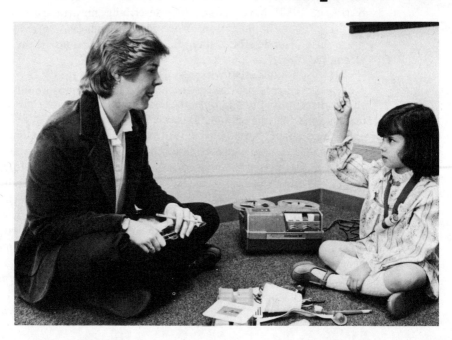

It goes without saying that planning a remediation program must begin with a careful and specific delineation of how the child's articulation differs from the speech of mature adults in his community. A basic tenet of phonology is that these differences will exhibit broad patterns which may not be revealed by the traditional method of articulation testing which assesses individual phonemes without regard to context. That is, phonological problems similarly affect whole classes, positions, and groupings of sounds. The goal of phonological analysis is to identify these deficient patterns.

Two primary changes from traditional assessment procedures are required for this kind of analysis. First, the entire word must be observed, as some misarticulations are related to sequential position, or to what occurs in the rest of the word; and second, differences must be described through some means that reveal their systematicity, rather than simply noting individual substitutions, as /k/→/t/. Several methods have been developed for accomplishing the latter goal. Influenced by the approach to generative phonology of Chomsky & Halle (1968), some speech-language pathologists (e.g., Compton, 1970, 1975; Oller, 1973) experimented with distinctive feature rule statements. Others (e.g., McReynolds & Huston, 1971; Costello & Onstine, 1976) totaled the percentage of incorrect usage of each feature. In another approach, phonological rules stated in phonemic terms were utilized (Smith, 1973; Compton, 1975). More recently, many phonologists (e.g., Edwards & Bernhardt, 1973; Ingram, 1976; Shriberg, 1980) have found that describing misarticulations as resulting from simplification processes (Stampe, 1969) provides a more easily understood identification of variations from the attempted target.

Certain phonologists (Weismer, Dinnsen & Elbert, 1981) reject process statements because of the implied assumptions about the child's perception. For example, the term, Final Consonant Deletion, may suggest that the child actually perceived the presence of a final consonant which he omits, which sometimes has been impossible to prove. The issue lies, it seems, in the semantics of the term, "process," which suggests action taken or choice made by the child. Certainly, a great deal more research is needed on how children perceive adult speech, how they internally organize the acoustic signals they perceive, and how their surface forms relate to their internal organization of these signals before we can make positive statements concerning the cause of a child's phonological system. In the meantime, process statements are useful in planning remediation even if they are looked upon as simply descriptions of observed deficient patterns. That is, there can be no argument when postvocalic consonants are omitted/deleted/absent that they need to be added for greater intelligibility. Or, if the child uses only one of the segments of a cluster, or fails ever to use the feature stridency, or repeats the same phoneme twice in a word instead of correctly using two different ones, that we need to concentrate on eliminating these simplifications, whatever caused them. We have not only described the child's surface system, but we have thereby identified removal of such conditions as remediation goals. In this volume, therefore, both terms, "phonological process" and "deficient pattern," will be used to identify frequent alternative substandard productions which occur across phonemes, while not implying any assumptions concerning what the child has perceived or "choices" that have been made. By contrast, the terms, "phonological pattern" and "target pattern," will identify what the child needs to develop to become more intelligible.

METHOD OF SAMPLING

The speech-language pathologist samples a child's speech in order to determine the deficient patterns. There is currently some difference of opinion as to whether this is more appropriately done by means of a conversational speech sample (as advocated, for example, by Shriberg & Kwiatkowski, 1980) or by a predetermined list of words elicited by requiring pictures or objects to be named. There is some doubt as to whether the method of sampling actually results in identification of different processes in the unintelligible child's productions. Bankson & Bernthal (1982) found that there was no statistical difference between the processes revealed by the single word responses and the delayed sentence imitations obtained by the Weiner (1978) test procedure. A study by Moss (1982) demonstrated that essentially the same processes were revealed in an unintelligible child's speech by either a connected speech sample or a single-word-elicitation procedure.

If the assessment is made for the purpose of planning remediation rather than observing the child's lexical or phonemic preferences, we believe there are important advantages in eliciting a carefully designed word list. First, all consonant phonemes and common sequences can be observed in various positions and contexts. Thus, it is possible to analyze both the array and extent of the deficient patterns the child would currently use, disallowing restrictions of his speaking vocabulary. Second, because the list of words is stable, readministration at a later time yields results which can be directly compared. Thus, the improvement can be clearly observed and accurately measured for accountability purposes. Third, and perhaps most important, only when the target word is known can some children's deviations be accurately determined. With highly unintelligible children, this is a critical consideration, since it may not be possible to recognize more than a few words without this knowledge.

It is possible to secure this broad sampling in a short time and to score it quickly, a condition which has obvious importance for the busy practitioner. Using *The Assessment of Phonological Processes* (Hodson, 1980), we typically transcribe the sample in less than 20 minutes and score it in approximately 30 minutes, after the child has gone. This instrument involves eliciting 55 spontaneous utterances as the child chooses and names three-dimensional stimuli. All American English phonemes are assessed at least twice—all of them prevocalically, as well as postvocalically, except /w, j, h/, for which only prevocalic productions are possible. In addition, 31 common consonant clusters are assessed, four of which are three-segment clusters.

Following the single-word elicitation, we record a sample of conversational speech. The words that can be identified in this sample are examined to see whether the processes vary from those in the single word sample. With unintelligible children they rarely vary. Most words in the conversational sample are impossible to analyze, however, because the targets cannot be identified.

METHOD OF ANALYSIS

Most clinicians are aware that the accuracy of phonological analysis cannot be assured unless the speech sample has been transcribed live and also recorded on audiotape to be studied later. As the children for whom this type of analysis is most necessary are highly unintelligible, it is often impossible to fully transcribe every word having heard it only once. In fact, even with repeated listening, examiners may find it difficult to ascertain exactly what sounds were uttered. Studying tapes, along with special attention to visual cues at the time of testing, provides the best possibility for a transcription upon which analysis can be confidently based.

Once the utterances have been transcribed as precisely as possible, each word is examined to identify and record all differences between the child's production and the adult target form. A single word's pronunciation may represent several different processes so each phonemic difference must be noted separately. For example, if *string* → /dwɪn/, four changes are apparent: the omission of /s/, /t/→/d/, /r/→/w/, and /ŋ/→/n/. Each difference is then labeled according to the specific type of modification which has occurred. In this example, changes are, respectively, Cluster Reduction and Stridency Deletion, Prevocalic Voicing, Liquid Gliding and Velar Fronting.

The 125 unintelligible children who provided the information reported in this volume demonstrated a wide array of deficient patterns. Some of these occurred with considerable frequency; others were quite rare. Sometimes a child used a process broadly; that is, he might at no time use postvocalic consonants. Another child might restrict this same process to specific sound classes, such as all obstruents, or perhaps just to one class of consonants, say, fricatives. It is important to describe exactly what the child does, since this identifies the focus of efficient remediation procedures.

The following section describes all of the broad deficient patterns and common sub-patterns which we have actually observed. These are listed in Table 1. Any one child will probably use but a limited number of the patterns here described, but the list will alert the reader to the variety of systematic deviations children may use. They fall into 10 major categories.

DEFICIENT PATTERNS WHICH HAVE BEEN OBSERVED

1. Omissions

a. *Syllables*. Omission of syllables may take two forms, or perhaps better stated, may exist at two levels. *Reduction to Monosyllables*: Replacing multisyllabic words with a single syllable, for example, *banana* → / bæ/. *Weak Syllable Deletion*: Omitting an unstressed syllable, as in *banana* → /nænə/, or *away* → /weɪ/. While the effect of Weak Syllable Deletion upon bisyllabic words also results in monosyllables, a distinction is made between the two deficient patterns because the former results in a less intelligible utterance: e.g., compare *banana* → /næ/ and *away* → /weɪ/.

b. *Consonant Clusters*. Clusters may be either partly or entirely omitted. *Cluster Reduction*: Omitting one or more segments of a cluster, for example, *string* → /trɪŋ/, /srɪŋ/, or /tɪŋ/. *Cluster Deletion*: Omission of the entire cluster, as when *string* → /ɪŋ/. Again, these two deficient patterns differ primarily in the extent of their influence on intelligibility.

Table 1 — *Outline of Deficient Patterns*

1. **Omissions**
   a. *Syllables*
      Reduction to monosyllables
      Weak syllable deletion
   b. *Consonant Clusters*
      Cluster reduction
      Cluster deletion
   c. *Consonant Singletons*
      Postvocalic
      Prevocalic

2. **Glottal replacements**
      Final
      Intervocalic

3. **Major phonemic substitutes**
   a. *Gliding*
      Liquids
      Fricatives
   b. *Vowelization*
      Syllabic liquids
      Postvocalic liquids
   c. *Stopping*
      Fricatives
      Sonorants
   d. *Affrication or deaffrication*
   e. *Major place substitutes*
      Fronting of Velars
      Backing
   f. *Minor place shifts*
      Shifting "th"
      Labialization
      Apicalization
      Palatalization
      Depalatalization

4. **Assimilations**
   a. *Velar*
   b. *Labial*
   c. *Nasal*
   d. *Alveolar*

5. **Miscellaneous deficient patterns**
   a. *Coalescence*
   b. *Metathesis*
   c. *Migration*
   d. *Reduplication*

6. **Idiosyncratic rules**

7. **Epenthesis**
   a. *Vowel additions*
   b. *Consonant additions*

8. **Voicing alterations**
   a. *Postvocalic devoicing*
   b. *Prevocalic voicing*
   c. *Prevocalic devoicing*
   d. *Postvocalic voicing*

9. **Vowel deviations**

10. **Non-phonemic alterations**
    a. *Tongue protrusion*
       Frontal lisp
       Dentalization
    b. *Lateralization*
    c. *Nasalization*
    d. *Pharyngealization
       or velarization*

Note that "cluster" is defined here as two or more consonants occurring consecutively in the same syllable, so that *Santa* → /tæta/ does not represent cluster reduction since /n/ and /t/ are in different syllables. Also, we do not define postvocalic liquids-plus-consonants as clusters, for the reason given in **3b**, below.

c. *Consonant Singletons.* The deletion of single consonants is usually limited to one of the two positions in which they can occur, although at a very low level of development a child might demonstrate both patterns simultaneously.

Postvocalic Singleton Omission: Deleting a single consonant following the vowel in a syllable, as *hat* → /hæ/. **Obstruents** (stops, fricatives and affricates) are the phonemes most frequently omitted. **Nasals** are less often affected by this process. Glides, of course, do not occur postvocalically, and postvocalic liquids are very seldom deleted, but are subject to another process, as will be seen later. (See Glossary for definitions of sound classes. A cross-listing of consonant sound classifications appears in Appendix A.)

Prevocalic Singleton Omission: Deleting a single consonant preceding a vowel in a syllable. **Obstruents**, again, are the class of phonemes most often omitted; for example, *hat* → /æt/ or *cow* → /aʊ/. **Sonorants** (nasals, liquids and glides), however, may also be affected, as in *yo-yo* → /oʊ oʊ/.

It should be noted that Consonant Singleton Omission may occur at the beginning or end of syllables whether or not the sounds are initial or final in words. Thus, the loss of /n/ in *Santa* → /tæ ta/ is Postvocalic Singleton Omission.

2. Glottal Replacements

The use of a glottal stop in place of a standard American English phoneme. This is recognized as a typical characteristic of speech of children with repaired cleft palates or palatal insufficiency. In addition, some children who are becoming aware that there should be final consonants in words, but who as yet do not have postvocalic consonants in their systems, produce glottal stops instead. The glottal stop may replace **Final** sounds, as in *hat* → /hæʔ/, or **Intervocalic** phonemes, as in *bottle* → /bɑʔo/. This process appears to be at a higher level of phonological acquisition than total omission of consonants, as the child is apparently marking the presence of a sound even though a typical phoneme is not produced. Nonetheless, a glottal stop is still a substandard production in American English and the consonant would need to be targeted.

3. Major Phonemic Substitutes

a. *Gliding:*   Substituting a glide for a sound in another class. **Liquid** gliding is the most common manifestation of this process; for example *red* → /wɛd/, or *light* → /jaɪt/. **Fricatives** also are occasionally replaced by glides, as when *fork* → /wɔɚk/.

b. *Vowelization:*   Substituting a vowel for a liquid, usually /ʊ, ɔ, o, ʌ, ə/. **Syllabic** liquids frequently are replaced in this way, as in *bottle* → /bato/, or *water* → /watʊ/. **Postvocalic** liquids may also be replaced by vowels, as seen when *chair* → /tʃɛʊ/, *doll* → /dao/ or *bell* → /bɛʊ/.

Note that when the child is unable to produce postvocalic liquid-plus-consonant sequences, as in *belt* or *card*, the liquid is typically replaced by a vowel, not a consonant, as would be likely in a prevocalic consonant-plus-liquid sequence (e.g., *black* → /bwæk/; *friend* → /fwɛnd/). We believe, therefore, that postvocalic liquid-plus-consonant sequences should not be classed with consonant clusters as defined in Section **1b**. The vowel used to replace the liquid is often /ʊ/ or /o/ (*belt* → /bɛʊt/or / bɛot/,or the preceeding vowel may be prolonged (*card* →/kɑːd/), often with an accompanying pitch shift.

c. *Stopping:*   Substituting stops for "non-stop" phonemes. **Fricatives** are the class of sounds most often replaced in this manner; e.g., *thumb* → /tʌm/, or *fork* → /pɔɚk/. **Sonorants** may also be stopped, as when *yo yo* → /doʊdo/, or *lie* → /daɪ/.

d. *Affrication or Deaffrication:*   Substituting an affricate for a non-affricate, or vice versa. Affrication may utilize the standard /tʃ, dʒ/ phonemes as replacements for continuant sounds, as in *shoe* → /tʃu/, but children sometimes use a non-standard affricate; e.g., *soap* → /tsoʊp/. Although the latter may represent a transition stage between /toʊp/ and /soʊp/, and therefore indicate progress in phonological acquisition, it should still be noted as a deficient pattern. Deaffrication replaces the target affricate with a continuant phoneme, as when *chair* → /ʃɛɚ/ or *jump* → /ʒʌmp/, or with a stop, as in *chair* → /tɛɚ/ or *jump* → /dʌmp/.

e. *Major Place Substitutions:* Substituting a phoneme in a non-adjacent place of constriction. In **Fronting of Velars**, the more common version of this deficient pattern, the sound used is farther forward than the target. Usually an alveolar sound is substituted, such as *key* → /ti/, or *go* → /doʊ/, although infrequently labial sounds may be used, as in *cow* → /paʊ/.

Backing is the reverse direction of place-shift, in which anterior sounds are replaced by back phonemes. The replacements are usually velars, although the glottals /h/ and /ʔ/ are sometimes used. Alveolars are the sounds most frequently backed, as when *two* → /ku/, but labials could be backed as well, as in *five* → /kaɪk/. Less frequently, the replacement may be even further back than velars; for example, *soap* → /hoʊp/.

f. *Minor Place Shifts:* Substituting a phoneme in an adjacent place of constriction. **Shifting "th"** is the most common version of this deficient pattern, where either a forward shift, **Labialization** (/θ/ → /f/; /ð/ → /v/), or a backward shift, **Apicalization** (/θ/ → /s/, /ð/ → /z/), occurs. Thus, *feather* → /fɛzɚ/ or /fɛvɚ/ and *thumb* → /sʌm/ or /fʌm/. **Palatalization**, in which alveolar sounds shift backward to become palatals, such as *soap* → /ʃoʊp/, and **Depalatalization**, which is a forward shift, as in *shoe* → /su/, are other types of Minor Place Shifts.

Minor Place Shifts are not especially damaging to intelligibility and therefore would be rated as lower in priority for remediation purposes than Major Place Shifts.

4. Assimilations

This is altering a phoneme so that it takes on a characteristic of another sound in the word or phrase, presumably due to the influence of that other sound. For example, when a child who correctly pronouncesd /t/ in *top* and *toe* says /kwʌk/ for *truck* it must be supposed that /t/ → /k/ because the velar feature was assimilated from the postvocalic /k/. Assimilation may affect an earlier sound in the word (regressive assimilation), as in the /kwʌk/ example, or a following one (progressive assimilation as seen in *pin* → /pɪm/.) It may result from the effect of a non-adjacent phoneme (non-contiguous assimilation), as was the case in /kwʌk/, or of an adjacent sound (contiguous assimilation), as when *spoon* → /fpun/.

Assimilation is usually identified by the feature which is duplicated. The most common types used by the unintelligible children we have analyzed are **Velar**, as already illustrated. **Labial** (*pin* → /pɪm/), **Nasal** (*thumb* → /nʌm/), and **Alveolar** (*foot*→/sʊt/). The examiner should be alert, however, to recognize other types of assimilation when they occur.

5. Miscellaneous Deficient Patterns

A number of other deficient patterns which reflect the effect of elements elsewhere in the word or phrase were also demonstrated by many of the children we observed.

a. *Coalescence:* Replacement of two adjacent phonemes by a single new one which retains features from both of the original phones; for example, in *spoon* → /fun/, /f/ combines the stridency of /s/ and the labial place of /p/.

b. *Metathesis:* Reversal of the position of two sounds, as in *ask* → /æks/ or *animals* → /æminəlz/. Reversal occurred over a greater distance when a child asked for "*push huppies.*"

c. *Migration*: Moving a phone to another position in the utterance, as in *quarter* → /kɔwɚ/.

d. *Reduplication:* Repeating a syllable or a sound in a word in place of all the others, as when *basket* → /bæbæ/, or *television* → /dɛdədɪdə/. Reduplication may be only partial, as when *television* → /dɛdəbɪdə/.

6. Idiosyncratic Rules

The utilization of a deficient pattern which does not fit into any of the classifications here described. For example, one child regularly used /w/ to initiate final syllables (e.g., *basket* → /bæwə/).

Unusual patterns such as these illustrate the fact that it is possible for children to develop what appear to be wholly unique rules. The examiner should not overlook these deficient patterns, since their very uniqueness may contribute to our difficulty in determining the child's target word.

7. Epenthesis

a. *Vowel Additions:*   Adding a vowel in a word. The **schwa** is sometimes inserted to separate the segments of a cluster, as when *black*→/bəlæk/. It has been suggested that this results from the child's inability to produce CCV sequences, so he reduces it to the simpler CVCV structure. Children with severe hearing impairment are apt to insert the schwa following stops if they have learned sounds in isolation.

In other instances, a final /i/ is added to create a **Diminutive Ending**, for example, *horse* → /hɔɚsi/, or *spoon* → /puni/. Since this pattern is very common in the speech of young normally-developing children and may have persisted as a result of adult attempts to talk at the child's level, it probably should not be looked upon as disordered.

b. *Consonant Additions:*   Inserting an extra consonant, sometimes with the effect of **Cluster Creation**, as when *fork* → /fwɔɚk/, or *ring* →/wɪŋk/, or sometimes simply an **Extra Singleton**, as in bear → /bɛjɚ/.

8. Voicing Alterations

a. *Postvocalic Devoicing:*   Replacing a voiced postvocalic consonant with a voiceless phoneme. This has been the most frequent pattern observed in this category, and probably should be considered "normal" for children as old as four years (Hodson & Paden, 1981); for example, *page*→/peɪtʃ/, or *nose*→/noʊs/. A prolongation of the vowel often accompanies the devoicing.

b. *Prevocalic Voicing:*   Replacing a voiceless prevocalic consonant with a voiced sound, as when *fork* → /bɔɚk/, or *two* → /du/.

c. *Prevocalic Devoicing:*   Replacing a voiced prevocalic consonant with a voiceless phone, as in *bee* → /pi/. This deficient pattern does not occur as often as Prevocalic Voicing.

d. *Postvocalic Voicing:*   Replacing a voiceless postvocalic consonant with a voiced sound. The rarest of Voicing Alterations, Postvocalic Voicing has been observed in such examples as *leaf* → /liv/.

9. Vowel Deviations

It is quite possible for vowel (and diphthong) alterations to occur without appreciably affecting intelligibility, as dialectical differences in American English attest. In fact, the examiner should be cautious about labeling as "vowel deviations" those variations which simply reflect the child's social or ethnic background. Some highly unintelligible children, however, exhibit clearly deficient vowel patterns. **Neutralization** is the most common of these, wherein all, or many vowels are reduced to one or two, most typically /ʌ/ or /ɑ/. Other deficient patterns result in the replacement of specific vowels, such as /ɛ/ (*bed* → /bɑd/ or /bʌd/).

10. Non-Phonemic Alterations

a. *Tongue Protrusion:*   A forward positioning for tongue-tip and/or blade consonants. This results in **Frontal Lisp** for the sibilants, most often /s/ and /z/, but sometimes the palatals (ʃ, ʒ, tʃ, dʒ/ as well, and **Dentalization** of /t, d, n, l/.

b. *Lateralization*:   Sound emission to the side(s) rather than centrally, which affects the sibilants primarily, but has been observed, though less often, in other sounds, including velar stops.

c. *Nasalization*: Nasal emission during the production of typically non-nasal sounds.   This affects vowels most often, although consonants infrequently are treated in this manner and not always as the result of palatal insufficiency; for example, we have heard what can best be described as a nasal snort, as in *smoke* → /h̃moʊk/.

d. *Pharyngealization or Velarization*: Production of consonants with a constriction in the velopharyngeal area.   This has been observed in some children's productions of /l/ and /s/.

Non-phonemic Alterations usually have little effect on intelligibility. While these alterations may need remediation if they persist, they would be of low priority in planning phonological remediation compared with most of the deviations previously described.

Since the description of deficient patterns is rather lengthy, the list is arrayed in outline form in Table 1 for more rapid reference. It should be remembered that a single child will use only a limited number of these patterns.   Some of them, you will recall, are opposite, such as Palatalization and Depalatalization, or Backing and Fronting, and both are not apt to occur for the same child. Some tend to block other patterns; that is, make it impossible for them to occur. Postvocalic Devoicing, for example, cannot occur if there is Postvocalic Singleton Omission, and there is little opportunity for Assimilation if the child produces only CV syllables (uses Cluster Reduction and Postvocalic Singleton Omission). For any one child, therefore, the list will be limited and perhaps no more than five or six will require intervention.

Each child, however, has his own more or less unique array of deficient patterns, among which there will be at least several very common ones that many unintelligible and younger normal children use. There may also be some which are found less frequently, and possibly there will be one that is unique. You—or we—may encounter a child who will demonstrate a totally different pattern than any reported here. In this case, describe exactly what is happening, noting the phonemes, positions, and contexts in which the deviation occurs, and label it with some descriptive/definitive term, just as was done in the above list.

In learning to use deficient patterns as the basis for analysis, it is helpful to first become familiar with the broad, common ones. Thereafter, it is not difficult to identify the remaining ones in a child's system.

EFFECTS OF DEFICIENT PATTERNS UPON SOUND CLASSES

The three classes of sounds which are most often deficient in samples of unintelligible speech are stridents, velars, and liquids. The most common alterations in these three classes are summarized below. In addition, changes that affect other general sound classes are described.

1. Stridents

The strident sounds /f, v, s, z, ʃ, ʒ, tʃ, dʒ/ are seldom produced appropriately by young unintelligible children; that is, Stridency Deletion is a common symptom of disordered phonology. However, stridency deletion may be observed in a number of different forms.

The most unintelligible children demonstrate Omission of stridents; that is, there is no replacement for strident phonemes. This may occur both when the sound is part of a cluster (Cluster Reduction) and when it is a singleton (Postvocalic or Prevocalic Singleton Omission).

Non-Strident Substitutes may be of several types. Stopping is the most frequent deficient pattern used (*saw* → /tɔ/; *five* → /paɪ/; *shoe* → /tu/). For some children, Non-Strident Continuants serve as replacements for strident phonemes. In one example of this, *soap* → /hoʊp/, backing has occurred, as well. Though rather infrequent, *soap* → /θoʊp/ represents another non-strident continuant replacement for the strident /s/. Care should be taken not to confuse the frontal lisp, /s̟/, which retains stridency, with the /θ/ substitution. Gliding has also been observed on occasion as a strategy for replacing stridents (*four* → /wɔɚ/). Deaffrication may affect the affricates (*chair* → /tɛɚ/).

2. Velars

Velars may be subject to Omission, perhaps in all instances or perhaps only in clusters. The most frequent process affecting them, however, is Fronting (*cow* → /taʊ/; *ring* → /rɪn/).

3. Liquids

Children treat prevocalic and postvocalic/syllabic liquids as two separate sound classes; that is, when they are unable to produce these target sounds, they tend to treat the two in different fashions.

Prevocalic Liquids: The deficient pattern most apt to occur is Gliding; that is, /l, r/ will be replaced by /j, w/. Another which is frequently seen is Omission, which may affect liquids, particularly in clusters (Cluster Reduction) and occasionally as singletons. Prevocalic liquids are often subject to Stopping by children who are highly unintelligible.

Postvocalic/Syllabic Liquids: The most common deficient pattern used with these sounds is Vowelization, although Omission has also been observed in these children, particularly when syllables are reduced.

4. Other Sonorants

Here we are concerned with glides and nasals, since liquids have already been discussed. This group, specifically /w, j, m, n, ŋ/, may be affected by Omission (Glide Omission; Nasal Omission) or may be replaced by non-sonorant substitutes, usually through Stopping.

5. Other Obstruents

In this group we include, first, the anterior stops /p, b, t, d/, which may be subject to Omission (usually Postvocalic Singleton Omission, although, less frequently, Prevocalic Singleton Omission) or, with some children, Backing. The remaining sounds, /θ, ð, h/, are most often affected by Stopping or Omission. Children whose phonological development is not as severely delayed may place-shift /θ/ and /ð/ by Labialization (replacement by /f, v/) or by Apicalization (replacement by /s, z/).

Of course, all consonants may be altered by Assimilation, Metathesis, Coalescence or any of the other deficient patterns mentioned in the previous section.

6. Vowels

If vowels are highly deviant, which has not been found to be common except in the speech of the profoundly hearing-impaired, they typically are affected by Neutralization. Other vowel changes which are not dialect based do not seem to fall into common patterns, but represent idiosyncracies on the part of the child.

In summary, whatever assessment instrument is used to analyze the articulation of the unintelligible child, the purpose is to identify specifically the deficient patterns which characterize it. Those we have observed among the children with whom we have worked have been described herein and illustrated in some detail. The more common deficient patterns have then been reviewed by identifying the manner in which phoneme classes typically have been affected. The need for observing whatever the child is doing systematically, even though it may not be included in the above list, must be emphasized. Describing the child's phonological disorder in terms of deficient patterns is the first step in determining where intervention is required.

EXERCISES

1. In Exercise 1, three productions of each of four words by different children have been transcribed. The top headings at the right identify the types of alterations which may occur. The *Omissions Only* section refers to consonants which are deleted, whether they are singletons or part of a cluster. Place a check in one of the first two boxes, *only* if a sound written at the top of the box is deleted or replaced by a glottal stop. The *Omissions or Substitutions* section calls attention to the alterations in sound classes. Place a check in these boxes if a sound is *either* omitted or replaced by a member outside the designated class. If all of the alterations in the word are not accounted for by Omission or Substitution, name the other deficient patterns in the *Assimilation* or *Other* columns. Note that a single misarticulation can show the effect of more than one deficient pattern, so that you may not have completed the analysis with one notation. See Appendix B, to verify your answers.

2. Exercise 2 shows the productions for eight target words by four five-year-old males. Although the samples are limited, several deficient patterns can be observed at least twice among each child's eight words. List these; then on the basis of the information about that child's system, predict which production, of those shown at the left, each child used for "thumb." Answers for Exercise 2 are also in Appendix B.

EXERCISES

Exercise 1 — *Identifying Phonological Processes.*

Productions	Omissions Only		Stridency Deletion	Omissions or Substitutions		Other Sonorants		Assimilations	Other
	Cluster Reduction	Singleton Obstruents		Velar Deviations	Liquid Deviations	Nasals	Glides		
soap → /toʊ/ /hoʊ/ /boʊp/	✕	/s/ /p/	/s/	✕	✕	✕	✕		
watch → /wɑt/ /ɑ/ /hɑʔ/		/tʃ/	/tʃ/	✕	✕	✕	/w/		
string → /twi/ /nɪn/ /kwɪŋ/	/str/	✕	/s/	/ŋ/	/r/	/ŋ/			
screw-driver → /tu daɪ bʊ/ /kwu gaɪ ɚ/ /pu bwɑɹ/	/skr/ /dr/	/v/	/s/ /v/	/k/	/r/ /r/ /ɚ/	✕	✕		

Exercise 2 — *Identifying Phonological Systems.*

Target	A (5;11)	J (5;7)	D (5;6)	T (5;0)
/fɔæk/	/bʌ/	/pɔuk/	/hɔu/	/ɔɪ?/
/nɔuz/	/mɔu/	/nɔus/	/nɔu/	/nɔud̥/
/glʌv/	/bʌ/	/dʌb/	/kʌ/	/dʌb̥/
/strɪŋ/	/nɪ/	/tɪŋ/	/hɪm/	/ɪn̥/
/kreɪ ənz/	/nɑ/	/teɪ ən/	/keɪ am/	/reɪ ənt/
/aɪs kjuːbz/	/aɪ t'u/	/aɪ tʌps/	/aɪ kjup/	/aɪ ud̥/
/skruː draɪ vəʳ/	/tu daɪ wu/	/tu daɪ bu/	/ku kau əʳ/	/u daɪ bu/
/tɛ lə vɪ ʒən/	/bɛ ə tɪ je/	/tɛ bə bɪ bən/	/tɛ ə bɪ wam/	/ɛl ə bɪ dən/
/θʌm/				

List below each process which is used at least twice by that child.

Who said
/hʌm/
/nʌm/
/ʌm/
/pʌm/
for the target /θʌm/?

(Fill in the predict-
ed production of
thumb for each
child.)

Chapter 3

Identifying Remediation Priorities

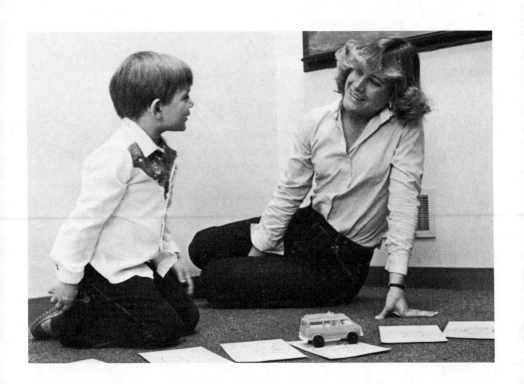

Identifying the deficient patterns which account for a child's misarticulations is essential, but it is only the first step in initiating a program of intervention. Unfortunately, most of the current literature in applied phonology does not go beyond this point. Speech-language pathologists need additional means for evaluating the individual client. Given the array of deficient patterns he evidences, how can the child's relative remediation requirements be determined? Does one child present a more or less urgent need for phonological intervention than another? The most immediate question, of course, is where should intervention begin? This chapter will address the issues of identifying priority clients and priority patterns.

On completion of a careful transcription of the words elicited from the child, comparison of the transcription with the adult model, and specification of the deficient pattern or patterns represented by each separate alteration from the target word, the unintelligible child's phonological system has been described. Many of the deficient patterns will have appeared in numerous words; some, however, will have occurred only once or twice. When thinking in terms of remediation priorities one concern might be the frequency with which each pattern appears. It could be assumed that those which occur with greater regularity are more damaging to the child's intelligibility than those with low incidence. Let us examine this supposition.

We can determine rather quickly the number of times each deficient pattern was utilized. Simply by counting the number of observations of each, we arrive at a frequency-of-occurrence total. Numerical totals can be misleading, however, because there will be more opportunities for some deficient patterns to occur than for others. For example, opportunities for Singleton Consonant Omission will exist in virtually all of the words the child has said, with Prevocalic Singleton Omission opportunities probably slightly exceeding those for Postvocalic Singleton Omission. Velar Fronting, however, can occur only when there is a velar target in the words. Thus, the number of occasions on which the child could front a velar will be considerably fewer than those on which he could omit a consonant singleton.

PERCENTAGE-OF-OCCURRENCE SCORES

A much more meaningful indication of the overall influence of each deficient pattern is obtained by determining the percentage of its occurrence. That is, if the total number of opportunities are counted and divided into the number of actual occurrences, this results in a percentage figure which makes it possible to observe the pervasiveness, or "strength" of each deficient pattern in the child's array. These percentages provide a better basis for the comparison of the influence of patterns. For example, if a child is observed to use Velar Fronting 24 times and Stridency Deletion 44 times, it might appear that Stridency Deletion is the more "serious" problem. When it is seen, however, that both numbers represent the use of the particular pattern on every opportunity afforded (100% occurrence), it is observed that both target behaviors are equally—and totally— lacking.

Percentage figures are easily computed for all deficient patterns whose opportunities can be counted. These include Syllable Deletion, Cluster Reduction, Stridency Deletion, etc. Possible occurrences for 10 basic processes have been counted for *The Assessment of Phonological Processes* and are shown in Exercise 3 at the end of this chapter. Counting opportunities may be rather difficult for a few, however, such as Metathesis, where it is probably impossible to determine all of the reversals which could occur, since these may affect not only pairs of consonants within a word, but also may involve consonants from elsewhere in the phrase. Likewise, opportunities for Glottal Replacement are difficult to count; and while we would expect Backing to affect only tongue tip/blade phonemes, a few of our clients backed labials, which would ordinarily not be considered to be Backing opportunities. Such deficient patterns as these, therefore, have to be assessed outside the percentage-of-occurrence framework.

If the speech sample elicited is a predetermined list of words as in Weiner (1978) and Hodson (1980), the number of opportunities for many deficient patterns can be counted for the entire word list and be available for quickly calculating the percentages for any child after the number of occurrences have been tallied. Hodson includes the number of opportunities for each basic process on her Summary form, and Weiner tallies it for each of his separate process evaluations, although not for the entire test. If a spontaneous speech sample is analyzed, the number of opportunities must be counted for each child individually if a percentage figure is to be derived. Since this would be rather tedious, the Ingram (1981) and Shriberg & Kwiatkowski (1980) assessment procedures suggest other methods for comparison.

INTERPRETING PERCENTAGE SCORES

Although percentage-of-occurrence scores compare the extent to which a child uses each deficient pattern, they do not, in themselves, indicate the extent of his phonological disorder. For example, a 20-month-old child whose speech is developing normally utilizes a number of simplifications described in the previous chapter, many of these at the 100% level, yet his speech would not be considered inappropriate. Obviously, the child must be compared with other children of the same age or stage of development in order to assess whether his articulation is, in fact, disordered.

Unfortunately, research on phonological acquisition by large numbers of normal children has been limited. No norms have been established as yet for ages at which various processes are suppressed. A study by Hodson & Paden (1981) of 60 normally developing four-year-olds indicates, however, that children of that age are not apt to use many major processes.

Table 2 shows the percentage-of-occurrence scores for basic deficient patterns for these children. Among them, only Liquid Deviations had mean scores of occurrence of over 7%, with /r, ɚ/ inadequacies appearing more frequently than those for /l/. These

Table 2 — *Percentage-of-Occurrence Means for Basic Deficient Patterns in Normal Four-year-olds (N = 60)*

Syllable Reduction	1
Cluster Reduction	6
Obstruent Singleton Omission	
Prevocalic	1
Postvocalic	1
Stridency Deletion	4
Velar Deviation	4
Liquid Deviation	
/l/	15
/r, ɚ/	20
Nasal Deviation	2
Glide Deviation	7

data suggest that the typical four-year-old uses a phonological system which is remarkably close to adult speech and therefore lend support to the contention that the child of that age who is difficult to understand needs intervention. But does every four-year-old with an articulation error need a phonological approach in remediation? Should remediation services by provided for any three-year-old whose speech appears to be delayed, or is there still enough time for them to develop "on their own?" Is a five-year-old with an "/r/-problem" a candidate for phonological intervention? These questions need to be answered.

DETERMINING PRIORITY CLIENTS

With limited clinic time available in comparison with numbers of children requiring training, speech-language pathologists often must make decisions concerning scheduling. We believe that not every child who needs articulation training requires the same amount of clinic time per week. Some can be served appropriately in groups, while for others, individual sessions are essential. For some, phonemically oriented remediation is adequate, while for others a phonological approach is much more expeditious.

In reaching such decisions, it is often helpful to have specific measures which objectively assess the child's relative needs. We have devised a formula for this purpose. While it must be considered tentative until it has been more extensively tested, it results in a Composite Phonological Deviancy Score, which reflects with considerable accuracy the comparative status of the 125 children in our program. In retrospect, it attests not only to their relative levels of intelligibility at the time of assessment, but also to the amount of clinic time required before dismissal. It also has provided an accurate index for grouping subsequent clients. We suspect that it would be useful in research for categorizing subjects for comparison within and across studies. The formula is derived using results obtained from *The Assessment of Phonological Processes* (Hodson, 1980).

Percentage-of-occurrence scores served as a starting point. When the mean scores for deficient patterns for the first 60 unintelligible children in our program (shown in Table 3) are compared with those of the 60 normal four-year-olds(shown in Table 2), it can be seen that higher scores reflect less adequate performance.

Table 3 — *Percentage-of-Occurrence Means for Basic Deficient Patterns in Unintelligible Children, Ages Three to Seven years (N = 60)*

Syllabic Reduction	7
Cluster Reduction	76
Obstruent Singleton Omission	
Prevocalic	10
Postvocalic	40
Stridency Deletion	72
Velar Deviation	55
Liquid Deviation	
/l/	81
/r, ɝ/	85
Nasal Deviation	22
Glide Deviation	38

For a single child, therefore, the mean of his percentage-of-occurrence scores provides a basic index of his articulation inadequacy when compared with those of other children. Certain other deficient patterns for which percentage scores cannot be determined because the number of opportunities is impossible to count likewise contribute to the child's total profile, however, and must be taken into account when assessing his need for remediation. The child's age is also a factor. These considerations were all included, therefore, in developing a formula for determining priority clients.

1. Determine the Average of Basic Deficient Patterns.

Ten deficient patterns were designated as basic because they occur commonly in the speech of unintelligible children and their pervasiveness can be measured by percentage-of-occurrence scores. These are listed in Tables 2 and 3. Once their percentages have been determined, the mean of the 10 scores can be calculated. This provides an initial indicator of the severity of the child's overall deviation. If this mean score is less than 15, we do not proceed further in calculations. This child is not a candidate for a phonological remediation approach. His misarticulations can be efficiently targeted by means of phonemically oriented training. If the mean score is greater than 15, proceed with the following steps.

2. Add Points for Other Critical Deficient Patterns.

As has previously been stated, children who are highly unintelligible usually demonstrate other deficient patterns for which percentage-of-occurrence scores are difficult or impossible to determine. If certain of these are used pervasively, they may have a profound effect upon the intelligibility of the child's speech. To reflect the influence of such patterns, therefore, a point is added to the previously computed average score for each three occurrences of any of the following: **Backing, Glottal Replacement, Stopping, Prevocalic Voicing, Prevocalic Devoicing, Reduplication, Assimilation, Metathesis, Epenthesis,** extensive **Vowel Deviations,** and any **Idiosyncratic Rules.** For example, if one of these patterns is used 15 times, 5 points are added to the mean score.

3. Add Age-Compensatory Points.

It is obvious that a level of phonological performance which might be entirely adequate for a two-year-old could constitute a severe disorder in an eight-year-old. Each age level beyond three years that a child's deficient patterns persist makes that child's needs for intervention more pressing, and consequently, the same score represents different levels of concern at different ages. One method often used in speech-language tests is "cut-off" scores or norms for ages. We have found both of these methods to be somewhat ineffective since there are often many additional factors which need to be considered. A method for reflecting the increasing urgency of the child's phonological inadequacy is simply to add compensatory points for age, as follows:

> 5 points for four-year-olds
> 10 points for five-year-olds
> 15 points for six-year-olds
> 20 points for seven-year-olds and older

The result of these calculations is a **Composite Phonological Deviancy Score**. The entire formula just described is illustrated in Table 4.

Table 4 — *Formula for deriving a Composite Phonological Deviancy Score based on results of* The Assessment *of Phonological Processes* **(Hodson, 1980).**

1. Determine percentage-of-occurrence score for *each basic deficient pattern.*

	No. of occurrences		No. of possible occurrences	Percentage-of-occurrence score
(Example	22	÷	44	= 50)

2. Obtain the mean of *ten basic deficient patterns.*

	Sum of 10 deficient pattern scores		No. of deficient patterns	Mean deficient pattern score
(Example:	620	÷	10	= 62)

3. Add points for *other deficient patterns* and for *age.*

(Example:	Mean pattern score	Points for other critical patterns*	Age compensatory points**
(Example:	62 +	4 +	10)

4. The resulting total is the *Composite Phonological Deviancy Score.*

(Example   =   76)

---

*   Add one point for each three occurrences of any other Level I and II patterns (identified on p. 39); e.g., if Prevocalic Voicing occurs 6 times (2 points); Glottal Replacement occurs 4 times (1 point); and Stopping occurs 5 times (1 point), the total points added is 4.

** Add 5 points for four-year-olds, 10 points for five-year-olds, 15 points for six-year-olds, and 20 points for seven-year-olds and older.

4. Determining Severity Interval To Ascertain Priorities.

The composite score thus derived not only can be compared with those of other potential clients, but also provides an independent index of the severity of the child's deviations. During the past six years, we have recorded the length of remediation time required, both in number of hours spent in the clinic and overall time span in months before dismissal. On this basis, grouping the composite scores into the following **Severity Intervals** may provide a means for identifying the child's level of priority for phonological remediation:

Composite Score	Severity Interval
24 and below	Mild
25-49	Moderate
50-74	Severe
75 and over	Profound

These intervals are meant to serve as indicators, rather than absolute divisions. The range within an interval should also be kept in mind. For example, a child with a low Moderate rating would rank lower than a high Moderate rating.

All children whose scores fall into the Moderate, Severe, or Profound Severity Intervals, clearly warrant phonological remediation. Those whose scores are in the Profound Severity Interval are obviously highest in priority. They typically require the longest period of time to become intelligible, mandate individual attention (rather than group), and need to receive the maximum number of hours per week which the speech-language pathologist's schedule allows. Children whose scores are in the Mild Severity Interval would be lowest priority for a phonological remediation approach and, in fact, the traditional phoneme-oriented articulation training procedures would probably be appropriate for training these children. (Needless to say, if a child has additional communicative disorders such as voice, fluency, or language, these would also need to be considered in setting priorities).

DETERMINING PRIORITY DEFICIENT PATTERNS

Having determined which children are *priority clients*, the next issue the speech-language pathologist would wish to address is which of the child's deficient patterns are highest in priority for remediation. We have arrived at an answer to this question by observing that the 125 children we have evaluated seemed to group themselves, regardless of age, into four general levels of intelligibility, which were labeled 0 to III, with Level 0 being the least intelligible. (Note that these Levels reflect only the intelligibility in communication, and are therefore not the same as the Severity Intervals, which estimate remediation time in that age is also included.) Deficient patterns which were found to be characteristic of each level were labeled Level I, Level II, etc., according to the level which they typically characterize. It should be made clear that most children evidence deficient patterns from more than one level. For example, a child using Level I patterns will also use Level II patterns.

Level III Patterns

Level III patterns do not seriously impair intelligibility, and, hence, we believe these to be lowest in priority for remediation. These are of three major types:

Non-phonemic Alterations
Tongue Protrusion, including both Frontal Lisp
and Dentalization

Lateralization

Major Phonemic Substitutes
Affrication or Deaffrication

Minor Place Shifts, including "th" Shifts, Palatalization
or Depalatalization

Voicing Alterations
Devoicing of Final Obstruents

Viewed from the perspective of which sound classes are in error, sibilants, alveolars, interdentals, and palatals, along with final voiced obstruents, are the classes which may not yet be produced accurately, although the deviations are very close to the targets. The phonemes are not omitted, but are altered in the ways listed.

Level II Patterns

These represent wider variance from the target than do Level III patterns. They are of two major types:

Omissions
Cluster Reduction

Strident phonemes, especially in clusters

Major Phonemic Substitutions
Stopping

Liquid Gliding

Vowelization

The sound classes affected are thus primarily stridents, which are usually either omitted or replaced by stops, and liquids, both prevocalic, which are typically replaced by glides or stops, and postvocalic/syllabic, which are Vowelized. These deficient patterns are likely to occur simultaneously; that is, a child who uses one will probably demonstrate all of them to some extent. Also, they are the ones we have most frequently observed among children we have evaluated. It would appear that this is the stage at which phonological development is most often halted, so that these deficient patterns perseverate long past the stage at which they would normally be suppressed. Liquid Gliding and Vowelization, in particular, may be so slow to disappear that they continue to exist along with Level III patterns.

Level I Patterns

These represent a varied group which may occur along with Level II patterns. That is, a child who is observed to use the Level II patterns may, in addition, demonstrate one or more of the following group, which in effect remove his productions even further from the target form. Likewise, children who are observed using any of the Level I patterns typically use all of the Level II patterns, either concurrently or as replacements when Level I patterns are eliminated.

Omissions
Syllables

Prevocalic Singletons, usually Obstruents,
  though sometimes Sonorants
Postvocalic Singletons, usually Obstruents,
  but sometimes Nasals
Cluster Deletion

Major Place Substitutes
Fronting of Velars

Backing

Glottal Replacement

Voicing Alterations
Prevocalic Voicing

Prevocalic Devoicing

Miscellaneous Patterns
Reduplication

Vowel Deviations

Idiosyncratic, or Child-Specific Rules

The sounds primarily affected are all obstruents except for the labials /p, b/, although even these might be omitted in some positions or altered in voicing. It will be seen that many of these are less intelligible deviations than Level II patterns. Cluster Deletion, for example, is more damaging than Cluster Reduction. Omitting singleton consonants decreases intelligibility more than reducing clusters. Stopping is easier to interpret if Backing or Fronting is not also affecting the production.

Level 0

This essentially consists of one overriding pattern:

Omissions
Obstruents

Liquids

Glides and Nasals; somewhat less frequently

In other words, children who utilize extensive Level 0 omissions produce vowels and sometimes glides and nasals, but virtually no other consonants. Consequently, they are seldom understood unless they use gestures. It goes without saying that Level 0 omissions represent the highest level of priority for remediation.

Assimilations, Metathesis, Epenthesis, Coalescence and Diminutive cannot be identified as to Level except by their surface form, which will vary depending upon what other patterns coexist. They may occur at all Levels except Level 0. The array of deficient patterns according to Levels is summarized in Table 5.

Table 5 — *Deficient Patterns According to Levels*

Level 0

Omissions

Obstruents and Liquids (less frequently, Glides and Nasals)

Level I

Omissions

Syllables

Prevocalic Singletons, usually Obstruents (sometimes Sonorants)

Postvocalic Singletons, usually Obstruents (sometimes Nasals)

Cluster Deletion

Major Place Substitutes

Fronting of Velars

Backing

Glottal Replacement

Voicing Alterations

Prevocalic Voicing

Prevocalic Devoicing

Miscellaneous Patterns

Reduplication

Vowel Deviations

Idiosyncratic (child-specific) rules

Level II

Omissions

Cluster Reduction

Strident phonemes, especially in clusters

Major Phonemic Substitutes

Stopping

Liquid Gliding

Vowelization

Level III

Non-phonemic Alterations

Tongue Protrusion (including both Frontal Lisp and Dentalization)

Lateralization

Major Phonemic Substitutes

Affrication or Deaffrication

Minor Place Shifts (including "th" Shifts, Palatalization or Depalatalization)

Voicing Alterations

Devoicing of Final Obstruents

As has been said previously, each child presents his own array of patterns, and it is quite likely that he will be using deficient patterns which span two or perhaps even three levels. Most lower level patterns, provided they are used extensively, are more damaging to intelligibility and therefore are of higher priority for remediation. Also, they will probably be more immediately responsive to intervention than those at a higher level. Consequently, Level I patterns which occur at more than 40% of their opportunities would usually have a higher priority than those at Level II, even if these are utilized at the 100% level.

Within each level, only those patterns which are scored at 40% occurrence or above are scrutinized to ascertain whether phonological intervention is indicated. If a deficient pattern is scored below 40% occurrence, it very likely will not require attention. It should be re-checked, however, during reassessment before a decision is made not to target it. At times, a deficient pattern will affect only a portion of its possible opportunities, but these may represent a high proportion of a particular position or phoneme type. For example, a child might evidence only, say, 50% occurrence of Velar Fronting when all of the velars are scored, yet 100% of the initial velars are fronted. In this case, prevocalic velars are rated high priority along with other Level I processes which score over 40% overall. Another example of high scoring on subdivisions within the pattern might be high Cluster Reduction on /l/-clusters only, when overall Cluster Reduction for other clusters shows a low percentage score. The examiner should take special care to look for such partial patterns which are used with high percentage.

In summary, speech-language pathologists whose caseloads are large may find the formula proposed in this chapter useful in ascertaining client priorities. The criteria suggested above not only make it possible to identify which clients are high in priority, but also to defend scheduling more clinic time for high priority clients and less for others, and individual time for those with high priority, with more group therapy for those with low priority. Also, the identification of high priority patterns suggests where intervention efforts will have the greatest impact upon the client's speech, not only at the outset of remediation, but also following periodic re-evaluations.

EXERCISE 3

Percentage-of-Occurrence Scores for basic deficient patterns and numbers of occurrences of other deficient patterns are presented for the four five-year-old male clients whose patterns were tentatively identified in Exercise 2 following Chapter 2. Using these data and following the steps outlined in this chapter, fill in the blanks to determine for each child his Composite Phonological Deviancy Score and identify the Severity Interval at which he falls. See Appendix B to verify your answers.

EXERCISE 3

Exercise 3 — *Determining Composite Phonological Deviancy Scores and Severity Intervals*

	A(5;11)	J(5;7)	D(5;6)	T(5;0)
Basic Deficient Patterns (with possible numbers of occurrences)		*Percentage of Occurrence*		
Syllable Reduction (21)	10	0	0	5
Cluster Reduction (35)	106*	86	97	131*
Obstruent Singleton Omission				
Prevocalic (38)	8	3	11	42
Postvocalic (30)	97	10	83	37
Stridency Deletion (44)	100	59	91	100
Velar Deviation (24)	100	54	46	100
Liquid Deviation				
/l/ (13)	92	100	85	92
/r, ɝ/ (26)	100	100	58	100
Nasal Deviation (19)	53	0	0	5
Glide Deviation (10)	60	30	10	50
Total	——	——	——	——
Average	——	——	——	——
Other Level I and II Patterns		*Frequency of Occurrence*		
Vowel Deviation	5 ——		5 ——	1
Prevocalic Voicing	14 ——			6 ——
Prevocalic Devoicing			5 ——	
Glottal Replacement	1		2	8 ——
Backing		3 ——	12 ——	
Stopping	14 ——	19 ——	5 ——	19 ——
Coalescence				1
Epenthesis		5 ——	1 ——	1
Metathesis	1	1	1	
Assimiliation				
Nasal	6 ——			
Velar			3 ——	
Labial	5 ——	6 ——	1	3 ——
Idiosyncratic Patterns				
Glide Syllable	13 ——		4	
Final /n, ŋ/→/m/			11	
Nasal Addition/Replacement				6 ——
Total Additional Pattern Points				
Percentage Average	——	——	——	——
Additional Pattern Points	——	——	——	——
Age Points for 5-year-olds	10	10	10	10
Total	——	——	——	——
Severity Intervals	————	————	————	————

* Percentages above 100 reflect Cluster Deletion as well as Cluster Reduction, since one instance of cluster reduction is tallied for each segment (sound) that is missing.

Chapter 4

Basic Remediation Concepts and Procedures

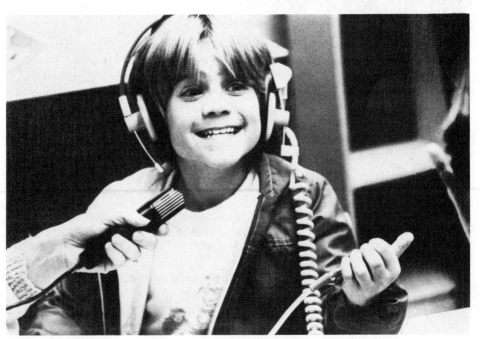

Identifying disordered articulation as phonologically based—that is, resulting from failure to replace the broad simplifications of early child phonology with the more complex structures of adult language—not only implies that assessment of the child's articulation should be in terms of the deficient patterns upon which he currently relies, but that remediation should focus on phonological *patterns* to be acquired rather than on isolated phonemes. In retrospect, it becomes apparent why the traditional phonemic approach to remediation usually required years of training for the unintelligible child. Teaching phonemes as separate units, often in unrelated sequences, and sometimes without regard for phonetic environment, resulted in piecemeal learning of surface forms. Little wonder that the unintelligible child was slow to sort these separate units into the underlying system that he was expected to acquire. Our phonological approach, by contrast, sets out to teach target patterns, utilizing surface forms (specific phonemes and sequences) as examples, and enables the child to later incorporate other phonemes and phoneme combinations into these patterns through generalization. Goals, both overall and immediate, are specified within this framework. In this chapter, the foundation upon which our approach to remediation is based will be explained.

UNDERLYING CONCEPTS

As knowledge concerning normal phonological development has expanded, it has become possible to utilize new insights into the way in which children typically acquire the adult sound system—along with some general knowledge which is not so new—toward facilitating remediation for the child who is phonologically disordered. We anticipate even more insight as such knowledge increases. For the time being, however, we have found it expeditious to be cognizant of the following principles when planning remediation.

1. Phonological Acquisition Is A Gradual Process

Ingram (1976) emphasized this principle noting, ". . .the child acquires a sound in time by stages." Dyson (1979), who tested 40 normally developing two-year-olds eight times at intervals of approximately three weeks over a period of about seven months, obtained data that strongly reinforces this observation. She found that, at this learning stage, a child's apparent acquisition of a phonological pattern as evidenced by its use in one word could not be used as a basis for predicting that the same pattern would be appropriately produced in another word. In fact, it was even impossible to predict that the same *substitute* for that pattern would appear in the rest of his words. Moreover, the correct production of a pattern in a word could not predict that the two-year-old child would say the word in that way at the next testing. She observed that many of these children vacillated among the correct and several incorrect forms, sometimes for several months, before the appropriate use of a pattern in a given word became consistent. In other words, many of the children seemed to require a rather long period of trying out or experimenting with the use of alternate patterns before they finally absorbed the target structure into their phonological systems. The fact that *all* of her subjects did not demonstrate an extended learning period may simply be due to the stage of development at which the individual child's testing occurred. For those whose form was consistently correct, the gradual learning may already have taken place, and for others it may not yet have begun.

As Ingram says, if acquisition is gradual in normal phonological development, "Should we expect the deviant child to be different?" Actually, speech-language pathologists have understood that it takes time for a child to absorb a new phoneme into his repertoire. On this basis, it previously seemed necessary to spend months drilling a child on a new sound, after he became aware of its auditory image and the articulatory gesture required for its production, in order to reach a designated criterion level. The question arises as to whether this "learning period" may simply be the usual time required by many children to "sort out" or internalize a new pattern into their sound systems, something which occurs without intervention in normal phonological development. Is it the basic acquisition of a pattern or its "internalization"—or both—in which the child needs assistance?

We therefore experimented with a program in which the unintelligible child was rather quickly and carefully provided with limited but successful experiences in producing a target pattern and then allowed to go about whatever internalizing, "sorting," experimenting or self-rehearsal of its use that children typically do on their own. Meanwhile, the clinician's efforts could be focused on introducing other new patterns. On returning to each of the original target patterns a few months later, we found that an accelerated review of each one which had not yet begun to emerge in spontaneous speech resulted in marked improvement in the child's use of that pattern. Thus, in a period that might have been spent supervising drill on one or two sounds, four or five broad target patterns had begun to emerge. It was on this basis that the concept of "cycle programming," which will be described in the next chapter, was developed.

2. Children With Normal Hearing Typically Acquire the Adult Sound System Primarily by Listening.

Although there is still much to be learned about what and how children perceive, the vast majority of them develop normal speech patterns with no adult assistance beyond auditory cues. Most parents do not instruct their children about "where to put their tongues," nor do they provide tactual indication for placement and production. While children who do not develop intelligible speech may need additional kinds of assistance, we believe the power of auditory stimulation should be exploited in remediation.

As early as 1939, Van Riper wrote about "the vast importance of ear training":

> The first step in remedial treatment of articulatory cases should be ear training... it is probably the most important tool in the clinician's kit. If the preliminary ear training is done well, little difficulty is experienced, even with the most severe cases. (pp. 123-124)

Most professionals heed this advice and include some listening experience at the outset when trying to establish new sound patterns. We have found that auditory stimulation is so productive, especially for preschoolers, that we incorporate it into every training session.

We also observed that our children appeared to be more aware of all of the characteristics of a modelled word if its production was somewhat amplified electronically. This observation seems in accordance with research findings by Elliott & Katz (1980) that, in order to perform at 100% accuracy in a task which required them to point to the correct picture representing a recorded word (e.g., dog), normal-hearing three-year-olds needed the stimuli presented in quiet at an intensity more than 25 dB higher than required by adults, even though the words were highly familiar to three-year-olds. Five- and ten-year-olds also required higher levels of intensity for 100% accurate performance, although not as high as three-year-olds. Furthermore, Elliott, Longinotti, Clifton, and Meyer (1981) reported that normal children required higher levels of intensity than adults in order to identify synthesized CVs (/ba, da, ga/) at 90% accuracy and, even more significantly, Clifton and Elliott (1982) found that articulation-impaired children with normal hearing required higher levels of intensity than their normal age-mates. This information has important implications for remediation which we utilize in our program, as will be described shortly.

3. As the Child Acquires New Speech Patterns, He Associates Kinesthetic With Auditory Sensations Which Enables Later Self-Monitoring.

Fairbanks (1954), in his model of the speech mechanism as a servo-system, described a speaker's ability to use correct sound patterns in connected speech as dependent upon continual self-monitoring, not only of the auditory signal we hear ourselves producing, but also of the kinesthetic sensations resulting from our generative and articulatory movements. Self-monitoring actually becomes antici-patory in the sense that initiating the wrong audible signal or wrong movement causes us to alter what we are doing sometimes even before the sound is actually uttered. In this way, we can often forestall inap-propriate utterances before they occur. In order for children to incor-porate a new pattern into their systems—that is, use it "sponta-neously"—they must properly "tune" these monitors. Since the sensors function simultaneously, the auditory signal and the kines-thetic sensation must correctly relate to each other.

We believe this concept has important implications for remediation. The child needs to learn what the phoneme "feels like" as well as what it sounds like. If he repeatedly makes a wrong articulatory gesture in response to the clinician's instructions to "Say /s/," the association between correct auditory image and incorrect kinesthetic sensation is fortified. For this reason, we place great emphasis on the importance of cuing the child for *correct* production of the target *pattern*, as will be described shortly. Establishment of a new pattern becomes habituated more rapidly if the monitoring system is tuned to enable the child to self-correct and eventually forestall an incorrect utterance.

4. Phonetic Environment Can Facilitate Correct Sound Production.

Practicing speech-language pathologists are well aware that children usually find it "easier" to produce a given sound in some words than in others. The position of the sound in the word and the phonemes which precede or follow it can have considerable influence upon the adequacy of the sound's production, particularly in the early stages of its emergence. It follows, therefore, that if words are selected for training which provide facilitating contexts for the target sounds, it will be considerably easier and faster to elicit the correct productions which are essential for establishing the child's accurate kinesthetic image of the sound described in the preceding section.

Predictions of appropriate contexts can be made from observing those phonetic environments in which normal-speaking children typically produce the sound first, and those in which children with articulation deficits pronounce it most adequately. Scattered information on certain sounds is available in the literature on both of these aspects. Several researchers (e.g., Edwards, 1978; Compton, 1977), have reported that in normal phonological development, singleton fricatives appear first in the word-final position. Dyson (1979) reported that in her 40 normally developing two-year-olds, velars were produced more often adjacent to back than to front vowels. Children with /r/ errors were found by Swisher (1973) to have more correct /r/ responses following /d/ and /g/ than following /f/ or /p/ while Gallagher & Shriner (1975a, b) found higher rates of correct /s/ production preceeding /t/ or /d/ than preceeding vowels. Kent (1982) provides an excellent summary of much of this information. Such research observations must be tested, of course, for clinical applicability. Experience with phonologically disordered children can provide additional clues for selection of words to facilitate correct production.

Commensurate with our goal of enabling the child to experience the desired target as rapidly as possible, careful preselection of practice words is of utmost importance. Although this is an area in which we need still more information, a later selection will provide specific suggestions for predicting facilitating words.

5. Children Tend To Generalize New Articulation Skills To Other Targets.

When learning third person present tense of verbs, young children very easily absorb the rule of adding -s to the first person forms and apply it, usually without instruction, to most verbs they use. Indeed, many children over-generalize this rule so that it is not uncommon for inappropriate forms such as *he bes* and *she gots* to occur for a brief time. Similarly, speech-language pathologists who have worked with a child on the /t/ for /s/ substitution have often observed upon re-evaluation that previous /p/ for /f/ and /d/ for /z/ substitutions are no longer frequent in the child's speech. What appears to be

"spontaneous improvement" is most likely an indication of generalization to other members of the same phonemic class. McReynolds
and Bennett (1972) tested this hypothesis in a highly controlled study
and provided strong evidence that features generalized across several
phonemes although there had been training on only one phoneme.
Weiner (1981) observed the effects of generalization in two clients
and noted that it affected non-treated words more rapidly for some
processes than for others. In addition, he found that generalization
continued with both clients after formal clinic sessions had ceased.

The tendency to generalize can provide important assistance in
the remediation process, and we program in such a way as to take
advantage of this tendency. It is not necessary to teach all of the
phonemes that are included in a pattern. We focus on only a few and
allow time for generalization to take place to the extent that the
particular child applies it. Younger children typically have been found
to generalize more readily. Older ones seem to be more rigid in their
error patterns and need more assistance in applying a new one.

All of the five concepts just described have influenced our
remediation procedures in ways that will be recognized in the
following and in Chapter 5.

BASIC PROCEDURES

Since their earliest attempts at improving articulation, members of
our profession have approached the remediation of articulation with
the understanding that two basic procedures are essential: making
the client aware of the characteristics of the target sound or sound
combinations; and eliciting a sufficient number of correct productions of the target so that the child becomes able to utilize this ability
in spontaneous speech. In other words, remediation has always
focused on stimulation and production, and our approach to phonological remediation does not change this basic focus. We do, however,
use some different techniques, and we advocate some different stan-
dards in achieving goals than have been common in traditional
programming.

Stimulation

Auditory. Since they are the "natural," and primary, cues through
which the great majority of children acquire the sound system of
language, it would seem logical that the child who is phonologically
disordered might also profit from attending to the audible
characteristics of sounds. Although it might be argued that the

unintelligible child has probably had as much opportunity to hear language as the typical child, it may be that these children simply require more—or perhaps more concentrated or emphasized—auditory stimulation than usual. Or, in light of Clifton and Elliott's previously cited findings, the child with disordered phonology may experience extreme difficulty perceiving sounds without some amplification. Furthermore, a higher than chance proportion of the 125 children in our phonology program had histories of otitis media. The mild or fluctuant hearing loss that commonly accompanies this condition may have been a factor in hindering their hearing of sound patterns at a critical period in speech development.

For whatever reason, we have found that with unintelligible children, "auditory bombardment"—listening to numerous repetitions at a low level of amplification of words containing the target sound or sequence—produced awareness that was not achieved through regular listening, nor by other methods. With Van Riper, we have found that ear training is "the most important tool in the clinician's kit." In our program, however, we do not restrict it to a "preliminary" activity. Approximately two minutes of auditory bombardment are provided at the beginning and end of *every* session, in the following manner:

While the child is engaged in some quiet hand activity, such as working with Play-Doh or coloring, the clinician reads words containing the target for that session; e.g., final /p/, prevocalic /st/, or prevocalic /l/. These words should be ones the child understands, but, as he will not be asked to repeat them, they need not be carefully selected. The words should be read distinctly, but not exaggerated. The child wears earphones connected to some device that will produce low amplification. Depending on what is available in the particular facility, this may be any one of the brands of auditory training units which has an external microphone, or even a tape recorder into which an external microphone and earphones are plugged.

Auditory training units, it should be remembered, are designed for use by persons with impaired hearing and are capable of producing high amplification. Caution must be taken to keep the level minimal and to prevent feedback blasts in order to avoid any possible damage to the child's hearing mechanism. The clinician should take the precaution of testing the level by putting on the earphones and speaking a few words into the microphone at the loudness she intends to use before placing the earphones on the child. And, of course, she should turn the machine off before taking the earphone off herself or the child to avoid feedback. Properly used, however, amplification has proved to be a remarkably efficient means for helping the child focus on the sound pattern. The earphones shut out other noise in the room which might distract; the low amplification then emphasizes the sound characteristics, and figure-ground contrast is aided. When the clinician attempts to do this without amplification, the exaggeration that often results defeats the purpose, and the child may attend to other noises in the environment rather than the target sounds.

Auditory training units are rather expensive and if the budget does not permit their purchase, a tape recorder may serve. In using a tape recorder for amplification, operate the instrument in the "Record" mode (there need not be a tape in the machine). Again, put the earphones on yourself, and speak a few words directly into the microphone to insure that the level is well within the comfort range. Use this same setting as the child listens.

Tactual. Many children, in the case of some if not all phonemes, seem to require additional types of stimulation in order to develop awareness of the target pattern. While we believe that auditory stimulation should receive primary emphasis as a means of developing sound awareness, we use tactual cues as supplements when first presenting the new target, and fade them out as the child gains facility. Tactual cues are simply ways in which the child can, through feeling, gain additional information about the image of the target. They may take any form which seems to work with the particular child. For example, to give the impression of an /s/ + stop cluster, the clinician may draw her finger up the child's bare arm while saying /s/ and tap it lightly as she releases the /t/, thus calling attention to the continuancy of /s/ and the quick burst of /t/. To indicate alveolar placement as in /d/ or /t/, a finger tapped lightly on the upper lip may be helpful, while for velar /k/ or /g/ the thumb and forefinger placed on the throat at the base of the tongue may induce the desired place of constriction. These latter two suggestions are derived from a system developed by Young and Stinchfield in the 1930s, called "Moto-kinesthetic speech training" (Young & Hawk, 1955) which relies heavily on tactual cues. Many other tactual indicators of placement and gesture are described in their book. The imaginative speech-language pathologist will devise many additions to this list when prompted by the needs of the child, since they are easy to invent if one concentrates on the characterisitcs of the sound on which the child's attention is to be focused.

One auditory training unit includes a small vibrator attachment which the child can hold in his palm, or it can be held on the back of his hand or on his bare knee or arm. Speaking a strident sound, such as /s/ or /ʃ/, into the microphone produces an easily sensed tactual image of a continuant, noisy sound, particularly in contrast with a stop, which is felt as a quick pulse. We have observed that many children produce certain desired targets much more readily when they receive this combined auditory and tactual stimulation.

Visual. Speech-language pathologists learned long ago that visual stimulation can be an effective supplemental cue. Thus, "Watch me," or "Look what my lips are doing," or "Look in the mirror and put your tongue where mine is," are common instructions given to children when teaching sounds. These cues are also employed in our program whenever a child seems to need them.

In summary, we rely primarily and heavily on auditory stimulation, believing that it is, overall, the most advantageous method for cuing the child. It is not only the primary type of stimulation used, but we continued to use it all through the child's phonology program. We also use tactual and visual stimulation as needed to elicit the targets. The cues, including models, are gradually faded out, however, as the child evidences awareness of the image of the sound and becomes readily able to produce it in the target words.

Production

Hand-in-hand with the development of awareness of a new pattern, the child needs experience in producing it, for he must start setting up the kinesthetic as well as auditory images in his multi-faceted sensor system for eventual self-monitoring. Here we strongly emphasize the importance of his saying the sound or sequence as correctly as possible (though not necessarily the whole word), so that his monitors become appropriately synchronized. An incorrect production may reinforce the wrong kinesthetic sensations for the sound that was modeled. Five good /s/ productions, for example, help establish the appropriate relationship; forty attempts at /s/ of which 15 are produced as /t/ or /ʃ/, probably does as much to reinforce the deficient pattern as to establish the target skill. Therefore, we do not specify the goal of a clinic session in terms of the *number* of attempts at the sound to be elicited from the child. We do not *count* his attempts. We do not *chart* the number of productions from session to session.

Rather, our planning concentrates heavily on ways of facilitating the child's correct utterance of the day's target sound or sequence. Two methods which help the child achieve success are careful selection of the practice words he will be asked to say, and utilization of auditory and tactual cues as needed.

In selecting the day's target words, it is imperative to consider the phonetic environment provided for the sound. Certain adjacent phonemes are facilitating for some classes of sounds, as was described under Underlying Concept 4. Words should be chosen to take advantage of such likely predeterminants of success. Detailed suggestions for these kinds of words are provided later in this book. On the other hand, assimilation effects which may deter correct production should be carefully avoided, such as asking a child who has Velar Fronting to say "cut." Even though the back vowel /ʌ/ is a facilitating environment for velars, the final /t/ makes it likely that the unintelligible child will say /tʌt/.

Cues which help the child focus on the desired pattern may be semantic as well as tactual and visual. For example, if *boat* is used as a word for eliciting postvocalic /t/, before the child is asked to name the picture, we often ask, "Is this /boʊ/ or /boʊt/?" If /st/ clusters are the day's target, when presenting a picture to elicit *stack*, we might ask, "It is /tæk/ or /stæk/?"

Experience has demonstrated that for children whose phonological development is severely or profoundly delayed, the task of producing the contrast between new and old patterns (for example, Velar /k/ vs. Alveolar /t/) in minimal pair words, as suggested by Blache, Parsons, & Humphreys (1981) and Weiner (1981), among others, is too difficult in the early stages of training for the child at the Severe or Profound Severity Interval. Semantic differences can be explained at this stage, but the focus is on the new target. We do frequently incorporate one "foil" word for the more advanced youngsters. For example, when /st/ words are being targeted, we might have a picture of a *top* along with *stop*, and explain that the "s" is necessary to make the difference between the two words. As unintelligible children progress and as they evidence greater facility with the new patterns, minimal pair contrasting can be used successfully, but premature use seems to result in confusion and failure. The purpose of production practice is to develop an articulation capability and a new kinesthetic image option.

In summary, we believe that remediation procedures should stress both stimulation for the target sound or sequence and practice in its correct production. While these are the same principles which speech-language pathologists typically follow, our approach has been influenced by five underlying concepts which markedly alter traditional methods. Time is allowed for the gradualness of pattern acquisition; auditory stimulation with increased intensity of the signal is heavily relied on; eliciting correct production from the outset is considered to be essential for establishing kinesthetic monitoring; careful selection of phonetic environment to facilitate correct production is therefore stressed; and we take advantage of children's tendencies to generalize new skills. The specifics for programming remediation of these basics are set forth in the next chapter.

Chapter 5

Programming Remediation

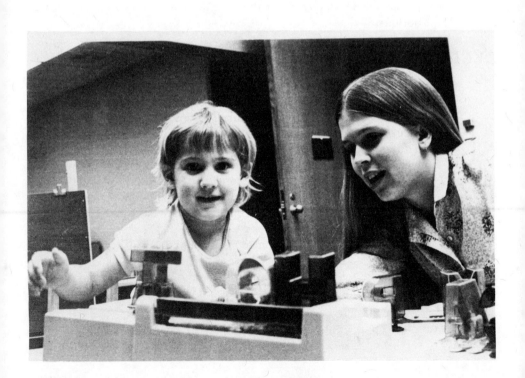

The traditional approach to articulation remediation has been that the child needed to be trained to produce virtually every sound which he did not say appropriately, according to singleton consonant acquisition norms (for example, Templin, 1957), and that drill on each sound should continue until the child uttered it correctly every time or at least to a predetermined high criterion level. Our approach to remediation differs from this procedure in two essential ways. First, we do not work on every error sound. We take advantage of children's ability to do some generalization and target only enough phonemes within a pattern to activate this tendency. The number of sounds requiring direct teaching seems to increase with the age of the child; that is, younger children typically generalize more readily than older ones. Second, we concentrate on facilitating phonological pattern emergence, rather than on "drill" or on "perfecting phoneme segments." Since absorption of a pattern into the child's system is something he can and usually will accomplish by himself, albeit gradually, we use the time this is happening to facilitate other phonological patterns.

In this chapter, the overall plan by which we organize remediation will be described. Then the selection and ordering of phonological patterns necessitating training will be specified; followed by the method for determining the specific phonemes through which the patterns will be targeted. Finally, the format of a clinic session will be outlined.

CYCLES

Our overall remediation plan departs significantly from traditional methods. We do not continuously target the phonological pattern until it has reached a predetermined criterion. Rather, we restrict focusing on a pattern to only a few weeks (usually two to four), using a different phoneme or sequence each week. So, several patterns can be targeted inside of a "natural" time block; for example, a semester. This sequential targeting of several patterns within two to four months we call a **cycle**. Since most of our children had three to six patterns which needed to be targeted, all of their basic patterns could generally be targeted within a cycle.

The first presentation of a series of phonological patterns over such a period is referred to as Cycle One. In most cases, each pattern needs to be "re-cycled" one or more times. A second presentation of a series is therefore referred to as Cycle Two, a third as Cycle Three, and so on.

When the first cycle has been completed, we reevaluate to check whether any target patterns have been incorporated into the child's system to the degree that it needs no further targeting. Typically, very little carry-over is observed following the first cycle, although the new patterns are easier for the child to produce. The second cycle, then, is a review of the first, moving more rapidly through the phonemes used in the first cycle, along with a few additional targets. At the end of the second cycle, we reevaluate the child's performance once more. Usually a third cycle is necessary to provide additional training on those desired patterns for which insufficient improvement has been evidenced. The average number of cycles required is three, but some children need a fourth cycle. Five cycles were the most that were necessary for any child in our program.

Our primary requisite for dismissal was that the child be judged to be essentially intelligible by significant persons in his environment. Two other facts were also taken into account. There must be a substantial reduction of Percentage-of-Occurrence scores from pretest, and all basic patterns, including liquids, must be beginning to emerge. For the majority of our children, the posttest average of the 10 basic deficient patterns was, in fact, below 15, indicating that a phonological approach was no longer needed. While continued remediation was often recommended for a few Level III (intelligible) patterns, and perhaps for liquids, a more traditional one-phoneme-at-a-time approach could be utilized for these few remaining misarticulations.

The above description of the cycle format may be more readily visualized by example. Following the description of six clients in the next chapter, the complete array of cycles for these boys is shown. A second reading of the preceding section may be appropriate after Chapter 6 has been read in order to further clarify the concept of the cycle format.

Let us look at some of the details of this overall plan.

CYCLE LENGTH

Since we, ourselves, have used this plan only in the setting of a university speech clinic, it has been a matter of practicality that the length of the cycle be a semester. Not only is there an obvious time break of several weeks between these sessions, but in a training institution the student-clinicians move to other clients at the beginning of a new semester. In the discussion that follows, therefore, we will be describing cycles that were about 12 weeks in length, except for summer school, which allowed only six weeks.

There is no special magic in this time period, however. Cycle length is simply a period of several weeks which is a convenient block of time within the setting in which the remediation is taking place. The length of each cycle may be varied according to professional circumstances. In Chapter 7, specific comments will be made about cycle length and other adaptations that may be appropriate in the public school setting.

Session Length

The time length of the session we met with a client was also influenced by practical considerations. Because many of the children came from rather long distances, it was more economical for them to come only once a week. Training sessions were therefore scheduled for 90 minutes, with a 4- or 5-minute play-conversational break in the middle of the session outside the clinic room. "One session" in the following discussion refers to that amount of contact time. It could also be read, "one week." Again, adaptations in session length will be dictated in other environments. The total time of our session might be some guide, however, when the clinician determines how many sessions to spend on a given target. It has been found that approximately 60 minutes for a target phoneme per cycle seems adequate.

TARGET PATTERNS

The deficient patterns which are to be focused on within a cycle are, as has been said, the major Level I and Level II patterns which the child is using on at least 40% of the opportunities for their occurrence. The goal is to eliminate these deficient patterns.

If one wishes to think in the positive sense, the target pattern is the appropriate replacement for the deficient pattern; that is, Postvocalic Singleton Obstruent Omission is a *deficient* pattern which needs to be reduced, while the *desired* pattern to be targeted might be termed Inclusion of Postvocalic Singleton Obstruents. From either point of view, the intended result is the same.

Lower level patterns are higher priorities for remediation than are higher level patterns because they allow the child to experience immediate and tangible success. Therefore, lower level patterns which are at a strength of 40% or above would be the first goals if they are stimuable. Thus, if a child evidences Velar Fronting, Liquid Gliding, Stridency Deletion and Cluster Reduction, Velar Fronting (the only Level I pattern in the group) will usually be the first target in Cycle One, provided velars are stimuable.

TARGET PHONEMES

A desired pattern cannot be targeted in an abstract sense, but only through specific phonemes or phoneme sequences that it influences. Because asking a child to perform an articulation task which is contrary to his present system requires considerable effort and concentration on his part, it is advisable to teach the new pattern initially in terms of only one phoneme or sequence at a time. Therefore, at one clinic session, we would work toward facilitating emergence of a new pattern using only one phoneme during the first cycle. If Postvocalic Singleton Obstruent Omission were the target pattern, for example, during the first session in Cycle One we would use only one sound, say, /p/, in the postvocalic position.

During Cycle One, each pattern is targeted during two to four sessions, using a different phoneme or phoneme sequence each . session. To continue using Postvocalic Singleton Obstruent Omission as an example, if /p/ were used as the first phoneme through which to target this pattern, another phoneme such as /t/ or /k/ could be used the next session. These two sessions could complete our focus on that pattern for Cycle One, and we would then move on to the next pattern to be targeted.

Probing For Target Phonemes

The specific phoneme or phoneme sequences to be used in targeting a pattern are selected to facilitate the task for the particular child. There is no "cook book" list. While logical reasoning helps to suggest a group of phonemes that might be used, the essential concern is a sound for which that child is "ready;" that is, one which is relatively easy to elicit and therefore will facilitate the new pattern emergence.

To give an example, suppose once again that the target pattern is Postvocalic Singleton Obstruent Omission. It is logical that the child will find it easier to produce in the final position a member of one of the classes of phonemes already in his system than to target a new sound or sound class. Since he probably has some stops, one of these would seem to be the best target, and since children typically devoice postvocalic obstruents, it should be easier for him to produce a voiceless stop than a voiced one. Thus, our selection as a target phoneme will likely be /p/, /t/, or /k/. The final decision would depend on which is easiest to elicit. Therefore, before selecting the specific target phoneme we "probe"—stimulate the child with two or three final /p/ and final /t/ and/or final /k/ words. Whichever seems easiest to elicit becomes the first target sound.

Suggested Target Phonemes

The specific phoneme or phoneme sequence which will prove to be the target most easily acquired for a particular child is not always predictable. Children differ in their capabilities, of course. The following suggestions have emerged from our experience as the sounds which most frequently proved to be useful in targeting the major patterns.

Singleton Consonants. For the child who does not produce final consonants, final /p/ is usually easiest to elicit. When the child is a "backer," however, he typically experiences greater initial success with final /k/. By the same token, many of the "velar fronters" readily produce final /t/, but may not be able to produce final /k/ during Cycle One.

Some children omit final nasals as well as final obstruents. Such children may profit from a session of targeting final /m/ and a session on final /n/, or a combined session.

Although final consonant deletion was more common, a few of the children we saw omitted initial singleton consonants. Usually only certain classes were involved. In cases where obstruents are omitted, initial stops may be the most likely target. One girl omitted initial liquids and glides. She needed to learn to produce initial /w/. Another child omitted initial voiceless consonants. His targets were selected from among /p, t, f, s, ʃ, tʃ, k/.

Consonant-vowel-consonant. Some children can produce only final consonants (VC) in some words and only initial consonants (CV) in others. Such children need to target CVC for a session or two to establish this syllable shape in their repertoire. Words such as "pipe, pup, pop, peep" have proved to be successful target words. Two productions of the same sound, particularly the visually and tactually obvious /p/ seemed to facilitate the pattern.

Syllableness. Most of the children we saw produced multisyllabic words, although many deleted some weak syllables. There were a few children, however, whose output consisted mostly of monosyllables with only a few bisyllabic combinations. Hence, these children profited from targeting two-syllable equal-stress compound words for a session (e.g., cowboy, baseball, ice cream), followed by three- and four-syllable combinations the next session (cowboy hat, baseball bat). When "syllableness" was targeted, any phoneme productions were accepted. The criterion for "success" involved only the appropriate number of syllables.

Back-front contrast. Many of the children experienced difficulty producing velars. Some of these children could not produce a velar sound at all during Cycle One, even when lying on their backs on the floor. Probing and stimulation for "velarness" was conducted, but targeting was delayed until a later cycle when a velar could be elicited more easily.

Final /k/ was consistently easier to elicit than initial /k/ or /g/. Some children could produce final /k/, but not initial /k/ or /g/. (Final /g/ was never targeted because it is voiced.) For these children, initial velar presentations were postponed until a later cycle.

Several children who were unable to produce velars were stimuable for a palatal or glottal phoneme. Occasionally, /h/ or /tʃ/ was utilized for such children as targets to "break the anterior hold" (that is, to produce articulation of some sound other than labials and alveolars).

Target words for velar facilitation should not contain alveolars during Cycle One because of the potential for alveolar assimilation. Thus, words such as "coat" and "candy" should be avoided, where /k/ would be much more difficult than in "cow" and "car." For the child who fronts *both* prevocalically and postvocalically, words should not contain two velars, so "cake" and "coke" should not be used at first for such children. The "severe fronter" can only concentrate on either final or initial /k/, and therefore produces /t/ in the other position. Once the child has mastered postvocalic /k/, words such as "cake" and "coke" become good prevocalic target word choices because the regressive velar assimilation effect then tends to facilitate initial /k/.

The child who is a "backer" needs to learn to produce alveolars rather than velars. Most "backers" already produce labials. Final /t/ would need to be targeted and also initial /t/ and /d/. (Sometimes final /ts/ is easy for the "backer.") Whereas vowels such as /ɑ/ or /ʌ/ are the best environment for producing velars, /i/ and /ɪ/ have been found to be best for alveolar facilitation.

Stridency. Most young unintelligible children say "tand" for both *sand* and *stand*. When they attempt prevocalic singleton /s/ they show a tendency to say /s:tænd/ for *sand* and /s:toʊp/ for *soap*. Taking advantage of this tendency, it has been found that targeting /s/-clusters prior to /s/ singletons has been more expedient for teaching stridency to these children. Also, it saved time overall since it was unnecessary to teach these /s/-clusters later.

We observed that older unintelligible children who had had prior intervention which targeted prevocalic singleton /s/ before /s/-clusters typically said *sand* for both *sand* and *stand*. It is believed that this phenomenon was a result of their having been taught to delete the stop during articulation training which focused on /s/ before vowels. We have found that it is generally more appropriate to allow the stop to remain intact and to teach the unintelligible child to produce the /s/ preceding it. Asking the child to eradicate the stop at the same time the /s/ is being learned involves two difficult tasks, whereas producing /st/ involves only one—the addition of /s/. Furthermore, it has been found that prevocalic singleton /s/ can be taught much easier after /s/ productions have become acquired in clusters.

Many children find initial /s/-clusters easiest. The clusters which are typically probed for targeting are /sp/, /st/ (unless the child is a "backer"), /sk/ (unless the child is a "velar fronter"), /sm/ and /sn/ (unless the child has difficulty producing nasals). Some children find /sp/ to be easiest, but others have difficulty with this combination, especially if they have severe labial assimilation problems. Even though /st/ might be expected to be the easiest /s/-cluster target because of the "same place of articulation" aspect, it is surprisingly difficult for some children, especially the "backers." The /sk/ is usually easiest for these children. The /sw/ and /sl/ combinations are usually avoided during Cycle One. Initially, /sw/ seems to be one of the harder clusters for most children. Since most unintelligible children do not have liquids, /sl/ should be delayed until /l/ has become facile.

For other children, final stop-plus-/s/ is the easiest place to first elicit stridency. Since the use of final consonant-plus-/s/ clusters is common in language, it being a frequent plural form, this is an important skill to facilitate. Also, the semantic concept is rather easy to establish. It is the use of stridency that is the target; however, language structures such as plurals (e.g., *boats*), possessive (e.g., *Pat's*), and third person singular present tense verbs (e.g., *eats*), also profit from this focus.

Children who delete singleton consonants as well as clusters (e.g., say *an* for both *sand* and *stand*) obviously cannot target /s/-clusters until they have singleton consonants in their repertoire. Thus, a child would need to be able to say *top* before *stop* could be a target word.

Singleton prevocalic stridents /f, s, ʃ, tʃ/ are generally low in priority for Cycle One targets, and typically are not approached until later cycles. Preschool children may not need to target all stridents, since they often show considerable ability to generalize stridency to other strident phonemes and clusters. Older children seem to have less ability to generalize. However, the older children we saw usually produced singleton /f/ during assessment, probably because most had already targeted /f/ for a semester or two.

Liquids. Speech-language pathologists frequently postpone work on liquids, particularly /r/, because they are typically among the last sounds a child masters. Following the same philosophy, at first we did not target liquids until all of the other patterns had begun to emerge. Progress was then so limited on these sounds, however, that many of our children were dismissed from the Phonology Program without having achieved adequate /r/ production, so that some of them faced a rather lengthy period of /r/ remediation in school using a traditional approach.

We therefore experimented with introducing liquids in Cycle One along with the other major patterns. We found it much easier to elicit an approximation of /r/ in three- and four-year-olds, than in six- and seven-year-olds who had not previously targeted it. Progress was slow, but earlier liquid facilitation resulted in greater facility in these sounds by dismissal. In contrast with all other sound classes, we frequently had to accept approximations at the outset, rather than require correct productions.

We do not expect liquids to be produced perfectly during Cycle One. Rather, our goal is to suppress the gliding process. Usually we break the words apart and stress the vowel (i.e., rock is pronounced: /ɝ/, followed by a very brief pause, then /ɑːk/; that is, /ɝ/ /ɑːk/. In such an utterance, it is quite easy for the child to avoid /w/. Blending /r/ into the following /ɑ/ occurs in a later cycle after the liquids are a bit easier to produce, and after /w/ no longer intrudes.

Prevocalic liquids are usually targeted before postvocalic liquids. In fact, we believe it is not appropriate for a young unintelligible child to target postvocalic /l/ since their intelligible peers typically vowelize it (Hodson & Paden, 1981). Even though final "r" (/ɚ/) is usually not targeted, its stressed form, /ɝ/, is being stimulated, of course, when we break apart prevocalic /r/ words.

Children who could not readily imitate an /l/ in a word often profited from a week or two of home practice in tongue clicking independent of jaw movement. This was the only instance where we frequently found a need for oral exercises.

The vowels which facilitate liquid productions during Cycle One are /ʌ/ and /ɑ/. The vowels /u/ and /o/ are particularly to be avoided since they provide an environment conducive to /w/ productions. Likewise, words with labials (e.g., *robe*, *room*) are generally avoided in Cycle One because labial assimilation (/w/) is apt to result.

Consonant Clusters. Consonant clusters are facilitated along with stridents during Cycle One when initial or final /s/-clusters are targeted as described above. Liquid clusters are often incorporated in later cycles, and occasionally glide clusters, especially in three-consonant clusters (e.g., *square*).

More difficult /s/-cluster combinations such as medial and final /st/ and /sk/ (e.g., *basket* and *mask*) and three-consonant clusters are usually reserved for targets during the final cycles. The older unintelligible children usually needed to target every /s/-cluster combination, while the younger children demonstrated better ability to generalize once a few /s/-clusters had emerged.

Other Patterns. Although the preceding patterns were the ones most frequently targeted, there were others which needed to be included for individual children. Since there are many possibilities as to what these may be, it is difficult to give specific advice other than to be alert to less common patterns which have significant effects on a child's intelligibility and to select targets following the guidelines just discussed.

Certain deficient patterns tended to disappear without intervention as the major patterns were being facilitated. For example, prevocalic voicing, glottal replacement, reduplication and stopping typically decreased spontaneously as children developed their listening skills and as they learned new patterns which served as replacements. The case studies presented in the next chapter and the clients' scores shown in Appendix C support this premise. If prevocalic devoicing occurred, however, as it infrequently did, it was one pattern which sometimes needed targeting for a week or two at the end of the child's remediation program. As a whole, however, voicing contrasts were very low in priority for remediation targeting. For the most part, it was not necessary to target voicing aspects in children who had essentially normal hearing or only mild hearing losses.

TARGET WORDS FOR CYCLE ONE

Selection of target words for Cycle One production practice requires the most careful attention to the effects of phonetic environment. In Table 6 are shown two target words that we have found to be most successful for each of the major deficient patterns. These are not only the words we have used, of course, nor has every child experienced success with them. These words offer a starting point, however.

Table 6 — *Two suggested target words for patterns frequently targeted in Cycle One. The same words may serve for probing.**

Final Obstruents

Final /p/	rope, soap
Final /t/	hat, boat
Final /k/	lock, bike

Consonant-Vowel-Consonant

/p/-vowel-/p/	pipe, pop

Syllableness

Two-syllables	cowboy, baseball
Three-syllables	cowboy hat, baseball bat

Velars

Final /k/	rock, lock
Initial /k/	car, cow

Final /s/-clusters

/ts/	boats, hats
/ps/	ropes, cups
/ks/	books, bikes

Initial /s/-clusters

/sp/	spoon, spot
/st/	star, stop
/sm/	smoke, smile
/sn/	snake, snow
/sk/	sky, school

Liquids

Initial /l/	lock, log
Initial /r/	rock, rug

*This list does not imply that there are no other words which are appropriate, nor that all of these words or patterns are routinely targeted, and no others, in Cycle One.

These words can also serve as probes to determine what to target the next session. If a child cannot produce either of these representative target words even when slight amplification is used to emphasize the auditory model and when tactual and visual cues are provided, then it would be best to bypass that particular target until the next cycle.

STRUCTURE OF REMEDIATION SESSIONS

Our sessions with the child focus on the basic procedures, stimulation, and production. While the specific phonemes through which a pattern is targeted may vary from child to child and the practice activities are selected to match age level and interests, all sessions have the same general format.

Auditory Bombardment

The child is introduced to the session's target phoneme or sequence by simply listening for about two minutes while the clinician slowly reads about 15 words containing that target. She may repeat the words more than once or use them in sentences; for example, if the word is "shoe," she might read: "Shoe. You have brown shoes on today. They look like new shoes." (See Appendix D for suggested word lists.)

As previously described, a low level of amplification delivered through earphones is used to increase the child's focus. The listening words need not be within the child's present capability to articulate appropriately. He only listens; he must not repeat the words. While auditory stimulation continues throughout the session as the clinician cues the child on specific words or repeats a word when the child has said it, this first portion of the session involves listening only.

Production Practice

The child's practice for each session in Cycle One is based on two to five words which have been carefully chosen to facilitate correct utterance of that day's target phoneme or sequence as has been illustrated. The words should also be capable of being elicited through pictures or objects, since a variety of play activities will be needed to maintain the young child's interest. Very young children (two-year-olds and some three-year-olds) respond better to objects.

Most three- to six-year-olds like to draw their own pictures on 5"-x-8" index cards. The clinician writes the word on the card so that adults will be able to identify the picture. Older children who can read may prefer cards on which they have written the words. However, many children with severe speech disorders are also poor readers and work better with pictures than with written words.

Speech-language professionals sometimes find it difficult at first to accept the idea that it is productive to spend an entire clinic session using only two to five words for practice. It should be understood that we are teaching a basic production skill and the words are only vehicles. The comparative advantage of many correct productions, albeit in few words, over many partially correct or inappropriate attempts cannot be overemphasized. After the initial session of targeting a pattern, the cards from previous sessions on that particular pattern are also included in the practice so the number of words becomes larger.

First, the words are elicited a few times using whatever cues— auditory, tactual, visual, and/or modeling—are required for correct utterance. (It is only *essential*, of course, that the target pattern be correct. If, for example, the words contain an /r/, which is not the current target and which the child does not produce correctly yet, this is not an issue for the time being.) Then the cards or objects become the basis for three or four experiential-play activities which appeal to the child. These can be more active for younger children (See Appendix E for suggested activities), and more quiet for older youngsters (naming a card before taking a turn playing checkers). The child's interest level is maintained, particularly with three- and four-year-olds, by including several different activities in each session. If a child especially likes one of these, it is better to repeat the activity at another session than to continue until the child tires of it. For older children who are able to read, a few minutes of oral reading is incorporated into each session.

As has been emphasized, correct production is of more concern than the number of repetitions, but as many correct responses should be achieved as the activities can "naturally" generate. Modeling and cues are supplied as long as necessary, but are gradually faded out as the child improves in ability to utter the target appropriately. Most of the session is spent on these production activities which serve both to develop articulatory facility and to increase awareness of new kinesthetic options.

Probing

Before the session ends, the next target phoneme is selected on the basis of determining which of the appropriate targets within the pattern being or to be taught is easiest to elicit. If the child does not respond correctly to the clinician's modeling of these probe words, low amplification and tactual cuing may help draw attention to the desired sound. Overall rate of progress is accelerated if it is determined what skill the client is most ready to learn; difficult targets sometimes become easier after the child has made some interim progress.

Table 7 — *Sample Time Schedule for 50-minute Clinic Session for Early Childhood Clients*

1:00	Review preceding session's cards
1:03	Auditory bombardment of words for this session's target
1:05	Draw 2 to 5 picture cards (Clinician writes word on card)
1:10	Activity No. 1 (e.g., bowling),* using new picture cards only
1:17	Activity No. 2 (e.g., basketball) using preceding sessions' cards as well, if for same pattern
1:25	Play break (free conversation—perhaps leave the room)
1:30	Activity No. 3 (e.g., flashlight)
1:37	Activity No. 4 (e.g., fishing)
1:45	Probing to determine next session's target
1:47	Repeat auditory bombardment
1:50	Dismissal (give parent auditory bombardment word list and give cards to child)

*The activities mentioned here and others are described in Appendix E.

More Auditory Bombardment

The session ends with a re-reading by the speech-language pathologist of the "listening word list" used at the beginning of the session, again using slight amplification, while the child listens attentively.

A sample format for a clinic session, showing time allotments, can be found in Table 7.

Home Program

Progress was expedited when the child was provided some minimal daily practice. Since parents usually bring the children to the clinic and watch the session through a one-way mirror, they are aware of what we require in the child's performance, and it is easy to enlist their help in providing home practice. They are asked to read the 15-word "listening list" to the child once a day at some relaxed, quiet time. The cards used that week for production practice are also sent home for the child to name once a day. If the preceding week's target phoneme was within the same pattern (e.g., another final obstruent singleton, or another /s/ cluster) both sets of cards are used at home for naming. Only the new "listening list" is sent home, however.

Review

At the beginning of each session, the prior week's cards are reviewed. If the same pattern is to be targeted that day, these cards may be used along with the day's new ones for the second and ensuing practice activities, and both sets are sent home for the week's practice.

In summary, the remediation approach just described is based on successive cycles in which there is repeated facilitation for the child's basic patterns which need to be targeted. Such a procedure synchronizes with the gradualness of phonological acquisition and allows time for whatever generalization the child may do on his own. Furthermore, the whole system is being facilitated rather than a segment of it. Patterns are targeted in a progression dependent upon each child's individual abilities.

The structure of the clinic session makes maximum use of time available for stimulation and production practice with a variety of activities to maintain the child's interest. An illustration of the nature of cycles and how they were individualized to each child's needs will be provided in the next chapter.

Chapter 6

Case Studies

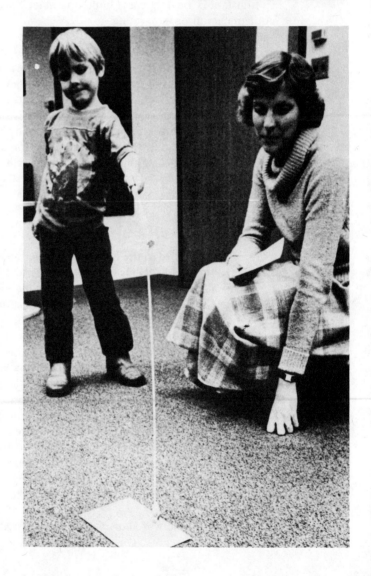

The programming plan described in the last chapter is more clearly visualized in terms of specific clients. For this purpose, the four males who were used as examples in Exercises 2 and 3 will be presented as case studies. Their phonological deficiencies will be identified and the cycles through which they progressed will be described in some detail. Two additional clients will be included in this chapter, one who demonstrated a very low level of phonological development at the time of admission to the program, and another who illustrates how maximum gains can be achieved when practical circumstances (in this case, limited contact time) require unusual adjustments in programming.

The remediation cycles followed in training each of these clients are arrayed in Table 8, which appears at the end of this chapter. This table will serve to demonstrate how the program differs when adapted to the needs of the client. There is no "cook book" order for selecting targets, since the clients' requirements and capabilities will differ even when the same deficient pattern is shared. Of the 125 clients involved in the program, no two followed the same cyclic progression. The pretest and posttest scores for all six clients can be found in Appendix C, along with their transcribed responses in the naming task.

JERRY (5;7)

Jerry first enrolled in the Phonology Program the summer before he entered first grade. He had received two previous years of speech remediation while attending an early childhood program and kindergarten. Audiological and otological histories indicated that Jerry had experienced recurrent otitis media. According to case history information, Jerry was above average in general functioning and in receptive language abilities. However, his academic progress reportedly was being hindered by his unintelligible speech patterns.

Results obtained from Jerry's phonological pretest evaluation (See Appendix C), indicated that his performance was at the Severe level. Jerry produced most final obstruents appropriately, including velars and stridents. His major deficient patterns included the following: Prevocalic Velar Fronting (which was his only consistent Level I pattern), Cluster Reduction, Stridency Deletion, Liquid Deviations, and Stopping. Jerry needed to target prevocalic velars, prevocalic consonant clusters, some strident phonemes, especially in clusters, and liquids.

Jerry's first cycle was short because it occurred during a summer session. The first week he targeted prevocalic /k/ in the words *cow* and *car* to facilitate emergence of prevocalic "velarness." He did not need to target postvocalic velars.

The second and third weeks, he targeted the two /s/-clusters, /sp/ and /st/, which were easiest for him to produce at that time. Jerry had already learned to produce initial singleton /s/ in his public school speech program, but he consistently omitted /s/ in prevocalic clusters. The fourth week of Cycle One, Jerry targeted initial /f/ (also to facilitate stridency). It was decided later that perhaps prevocalic /f/ should not have been targeted until Cycle Two. Although he could produce /f/, it did not seem to be as good a target for facilitating stridency in Cycle One as /s/-clusters were.

The last two weeks of Cycle One, Jerry received intervention on prevocalic /l/ and prevocalic /r/. It was not anticipated that he would produce perfect liquids at this stage; rather, the goal was to start some emergence of "liquidness," and to help him suppress his Stopping (substitution of the alveolar stop, /d/ for /l/) and Gliding (substitution of the glide, /w/ for /r/).

At the end of Cycle One, Jerry did not yet demonstrate any carry-over. However, productions of his practice targets required less effort on his part (fewer cues were required). Jerry returned once a week during the fall semester for his second cycle. He was also attending a first grade classroom, where reportedly he was experiencing considerable difficulty with phonics exercises.

During Cycle Two, Jerry again targeted prevocalic velars, stridency, consonant clusters, and liquids. Words which were a little more difficult for Jerry to produce (i.e., less facilitating phonetic environments) were added to his practice words. The first week of Cycle Two, Jerry targeted words with prevocalic /k/ and /g/, with no concern at this time about differentiating between /k/ and /g/, since the goal was "velarness" rather than "voicing."

During the next nine weeks of Cycle Two, Jerry targeted stridency and also some consonant clusters. Since /sp/ and /st/ had already been presented separately during Cycle One, they were "re-presented" during the same week in Cycle Two. The /sp/ and /st/ cards which had been drawn and practiced during Cycle One were retrieved for further practice, and also several new /sp/ and /st/ pictures were drawn and used in production practice activities. During the third week of Cycle Two, /sm/ was introduced.

For the first production practice activity each week, only the new picture cards were used. However, for the second and ensuing "games," the preceding week's picture cards were also utilized, providing they were compatible with the present week's target (i.e., within the same pattern). Thus, after /sm/ pictures were drawn, they were used exclusively during the first activities of the session, but for the next activities /sp/ and /st/ picture cards were also used. Pictures for /k/ target words were not used, since they were incompatible with the targets of stridency and clusters.

The target for the fourth week of Cycle Two was /sn/, followed by /sk/ the fifth week. Jerry demonstrated some spontaneous velar productions and for this reason was now able to target /sk/ without effort. During Week 6, Jerry used the *It's a ---* phrase to name items which did not contain /s/ in their names (e.g., *It's a door*). This was done to help him prepare for the next week's goal of naming his /s/-clusters using the *It's a ---* carrier phrase (e.g., *It's a spoon*). The only time phrases are routinely incorporated in our Phonology Program is when they are used with /s/-clusters to allow the child to experience success in producing two stridents in the same utterance, not for the purpose of using a carrier phrase, per se.

Jerry targeted some singleton strident phonemes during the next three weeks; final /tʃ/, final /f/, and initial /f/. Each of these singletons was presented and practiced separately for one week. The last two weeks of Cycle Two, prevocalic liquids were again targeted. Jerry demonstrated greater facility in producing them than in Cycle One, and was able to say more difficult words.

When Jerry returned six weeks later for the spring semester, his phonological assessment results and his spontaneous utterances demonstrated that he was using stridency and velars quite consistently, even in clusters. Also, singleton liquids were beginning to emerge.

It was decided that Jerry would continue in the Phonology Program for several more weeks in order to facilitate liquid clusters (including three-consonant clusters) and postvocalic /ɝ/. In addition, one week was spent on the affrication vs. deaffrication contrast in /ʃ/ and /tʃ/ minimal pair words.

Jerry's phonological posttest results (shown in Appendix C) provide information about his progress. Although there were still errors, Jerry's speech was judged to be essentially intelligible by his teachers and relatives. His mother reported that he was experiencing a great deal of success in his first grade reading, phonics, and spelling classes.

DANNY (5;6)

Danny also began his phonology program during a summer session. He had just completed a year of kindergarten. His relatives and teacher had reached a decision to have him repeat kindergarten because of his speech difficulties, even though intelligence testing had indicated that he was in the gifted range. Danny had received one year of speech remediation in his public school, with the targets being /p, b, m/.

Results from Danny's phonological pretest evaluation (See Appendix C) placed his performance in the upper portion of the Severe category (i.e., almost at the Profound level). He omitted most final consonants, except labials. In fact, he produced final /m/ in place of final /ŋ/ and /n/ (e.g., *string*→/hɪm/). The additional Level I pattern which Danny evidenced with regularity was Prevocalic Backing. However, Danny did produce some alveolars. It can be said that Danny demonstrated a preference for /k/ and /h/ prevocalically and /p/ and /m/ postvocalically, but that alveolars were emerging prevocalically. Postvocalic non-labial consonants were beginning to emerge, also. Danny's additional consistent Level I pattern was Prevocalic Devoicing, but this only affected /g/ (e.g., *gun*→/kʌm/).

Danny also evidenced Stridency Deletion, Cluster Reduction, Stopping, and Liquid Deviations. However, his word-final /ɚ/ productions were adequate. His primary targets were non-labial postvocalic consonants, stridency, consonant clusters, and prevocalic liquids. He targeted final /k/ the first week of Cycle One. The next four weeks he targeted stridency via final /ps/ followed by /ts/ for a week each, and then /sk/ and /sp/.

It is of interest to note some differences between Cycle One targets for Danny and Jerry. Whereas Jerry targeted initial /k/ because he lacked prevocalic velars, Danny targeted postvocalic /k/. (Danny already produced prevocalic /k/ acceptably and Jerry produced postvocalic /k/.) In addition, when the boys targeted initial /s/-clusters, Jerry targeted /sp/ and /st/, whereas Danny targeted /sk/ and /sp/. Danny's "preferred" word-initial sound was /k/ and so /sk/ was an easy target for him during Cycle One; whereas it was an impossible target for Jerry during Cycle One because of his Prevocalic Velar Fronting pattern.

When Danny targeted liquids during Cycle One, he had to bypass /l/. He could not produce it acceptably during the summer session. (He was only able to produce a pharyngealized /l/.) However, his final /ɚ/ seemed to help him produce good prevocalic /r/s. We have repeatedly observed that children who already produce /ɚ/ acquire /r/ much more easily than those who do not have this postvocalic sound. A number of our unintelligible children surprisingly used /ɚ/ when they had no other liquid in their repertoires.

Danny returned to the Phonology Program in the fall semester, while he was attending his second year of kindergarten. A major concern was to "get him ready" for first grade the following year. He began by targeting plurals as a whole. The model presented was final /s/ rather than final /z/. (Our experience has indicated that children are more likely to produce the strident feature of the plural form if /s/ is modeled, perhaps because stridency is more obvious when voicing is not present.)

The second week of Cycle Two, Danny "re-targeted" both /sk/ and /sp/. The third week he targeted /st/, and /sm/ and /sn/ were both presented the next week. Usually targets are presented singly at first. The first time a target is presented, it is the only one focused upon during that week. Danny, however, seemed quite capable of coping with both /sm/ and /sn/ at the same time without being confused during their first presentation. *It's a ---* phrases were utilized during weeks five and six. The next three weeks were spent targeting word-initial singleton strident phonemes, /s/, /f/, and /tʃ/.

Liquids were the focus during the last two weeks of Cycle Two. Danny had spent several weeks practicing "clicking" his tongue, i.e., moving the tongue tip up and down independently of jaw movement. Finally, he was able to produce initial /l/ and targeted it during the tenth week of Cycle Two. The last week Danny focused on /r/-clusters. By this time he was already producing most singleton /r/ words appropriately.

When Danny returned six weeks later for the spring semester, he demonstrated that he was spontaneously producing most singleton consonants correctly, including stridents and liquids, and that many consonant clusters were emerging. However, it was noted that there were several minor deficient patterns that were persisting. Danny regularly omitted medial consonants or substituted /w/ for them. In addition, it was noted that he rarely utilized /j/. Two other patterns were still persevering, prevocalic devoicing of /g/, and labializing of final nasals. It was decided that Danny would attend the Phonology Program once a month during the spring semester for some "clean-up" work.

The first lesson of Cycle Three was a "two-pronged" session with two quite different targets: /j/ and medial "consonantness." Essentially, he had two separate 45-minute lessons during the 90-minute session. His family and school clinician were given guidance to help

Danny master these targets during the month prior to his next visit.

The next month Danny focused on the rather difficult medial and final /st/ clusters (e.g., *Easter* and *first*), and the following month was spent on /l/-clusters. His last lesson was also divided in half. During the first part, minimal pairs contrasting final /n/ and final /m/ were presented (e.g., *cone* vs. *comb*). Minimal pairs contrasting prevocalic /k/ and /g/ (e.g., *come* vs. *gum*) were the focus of the second half.

Danny's phonological posttest results at age 6;5 are shown in Appendix C. He was dismissed from the university clinic at the end of the spring semester. During the fall semester, Danny's parents brought him back to the clinic for re-evaluation. Results of this phonological assessment are also included in Appendix C. It can be seen that Danny's phonological system continued to improve after his dismissal even though Danny received no additional speech programming. His speech still had some errors, but he was intelligible and reportedly was experiencing a great deal of success with his first grade lessons.

TIM (5;0)

Tim entered the Phonology Program the summer before he began kindergarten. He had been receiving intervention for two years in an itinerant speech program for pre-schoolers in his local school district.

Tim had a repaired cleft palate and a history of recurrent otitis media. PE tubes had been inserted nine times. Tim's speech mechanism was judged at this time by his cleft palate team to be adequate for speech purposes. Furthermore, he demonstrated during his initial phonological evaluation that he was able to produce all singleton consonants in isolation.

Results obtained from Tim's phonological pretest evaluation (shown in Appendix C) placed him in the Profound Severity Interval. The Level I patterns which Tim evidenced were Singleton Consonant Omission, particularly prevocalic voiceless obstruents, Cluster Deletion, Velar Fronting, and Glottal Replacement. He also demonstrated Stridency Deletion, Cluster Reduction, Stopping, and Liquid Deviations. One additional pattern which Tim used was Nasal Addition. The major patterns which Tim needed to develop were prevocalic voiceless consonants, velars, stridency, consonant clusters, and liquids.

Tim targeted six prevocalic voiceless consonants (/p, t, f, s, tʃ, ʃ/) during Cycle One. Prevocalic /k/, which overlapped two of his deficient patterns, Velar Deviations and Omission of Prevocalic Voiceless Obstruents, was not targeted because it was too difficult for him. Also, /θ/ was bypassed, as it has been deemed to be low in priority for highly unintelligible children.

Tim returned in the fall semester. The first two weeks, he targeted velars: final /k/ the first week and initial /g/ the second. During the next three weeks, the initial voiceless consonants were "re-targeted," two per week. The remaining seven weeks were focused on stridency. Here, Tim began by targeting final /ps/ and final /ts/, followed by plurals in general. It should be noted that Tim was not able to produce most initial /s/-clusters because he omitted prevocalic voiceless consonants. Jerry and Danny had both said *top* for *stop*, but Tim said *op*. He could readily produce word-final singletons and clusters, but the only initial /s/-clusters that were stimulable during the early cycles were those which involved /s/-plus-nasals. This may be related to the fact that nasals are usually fairly easy for children with repaired cleft palates.

All of the six prevocalic voiceless obstruents which had been presented during the first two cycles were presented together during the first week of Cycle Three. The next two weeks were spent on velars: prevocalic /g/ first and prevocalic /k/ next. (Final /k/ had begun to emerge in his spontaneous speech, and Tim for the first time was able to produce prevocalic /k/.)

During the next six weeks, stridency was targeted. Initial voiceless consonants were beginning to emerge in Tim's speech. He was therefore able to target initial /sp/ and /st/. In the next two weeks /ps/, /ts/, and plurals in general were "re-targeted." The *It's a ---* phrases were employed for the next two weeks.

Liquids were introduced the last two weeks of Cycle Three. Tim was, in fact, the first client for whom we tried facilitating /r/ before all of his other major patterns had emerged. When Tim returned after six weeks for summer school, he was producing /r/ appropriately in many spontaneous utterances.

During Tim's final cycle, he targeted the consonant clusters which were most difficult for him. Final /st/ was first, followed by combinations of /s/ and /k/. Coarticulation of these two phonemes seemed especially difficult for him, but he was finally able to produce them. The last two weeks, Tim targeted liquid clusters. If we had had one more week, we would have focused on three-consonant clusters.

Tim's phonological posttest results at age 6;1 are presented in Appendix C. He was dismissed from the Phonology Program after four cycles over a 13-month period. Tim continued receiving intervention in his public school with the focus being on voice quality and some Level III patterns. He was seen informally at the university clinic during the next two years. His phonological system continued to improve without any further targeting of singleton obstruents, velars, stridents, liquids, or consonant clusters. His parents reported that he was a high achiever in first and second grades. (Tim's case history and remediation program are presented in more detail in Hodson, Chin, Redmond & Simpson, in press.)

ALAN (5;11)

Alan entered the Phonology Program in the middle of a fall semester. He was in his third year of attendance in a special education cooperative school. It was believed that he could not succeed in a regular classroom because of the extent of his unintelligibility. Case history information revealed that Alan had had seizures and that he was receiving phenobarbitol and dilantin. In addition, Alan had a mild hearing loss.

Language measures indicated that Alan's receptive abilities were "within normal limits." In addition, Alan was highly verbal and he spoke rapidly, using lengthy utterances. It was completely impossible, however, to analyze his language samples.

Results obtained from Alan's phonological evaluation pretest (See Appendix C) placed him very high in the Profound category of severity. His major Level I deficient patterns were Omission of Final Singleton Obstruents, Velar Fronting, Prevocalic Voicing, and Postvocalic Cluster Deletion. Alan also evidenced Stridency Deletion, Cluster Reduction, Stopping, Liquid Deviations, and Nasal and Labial Assimilations. In addition, he had an idiosyncratic rule which involved initiating final syllables with a glide (e.g., *basket*→/bæwə/). The targets upon which Alan needed to focus were final obstruents, velars, stridency, liquids, and consonant clusters.

During the first two weeks, he targeted word-final voiceless stops to facilitate final obstruents. Final /p/ was easiest to elicit first; it was followed by final /t/. The third week we tried to facilitate "velarness" by targeting final /k/, but it was not a successful target, and we should not have targeted it for a whole week. We should only have stimulated it auditorially and tactually and by-passed targeting velars for the first cycle.

Stridency was targeted during the remaining five weeks of the semester. The first strident he was successful in producing occurred in the final /ts/ cluster. The next week, he was able to produce initial

/st/, followed by initial /sp/, /sm/, /sn/, one per week.

When Alan returned for the spring semester, he was still essentially unintelligible. It was noted, however, that final consonants were emerging in his spontaneous utterances.

During the first week of Cycle Two, Alan targeted final /k/ and was successful. He still could not produce an initial velar. He was stimulable for /h/, however, and that was targeted to help "break the anterior hold" (i.e., to produce some prevocalic "back" consonant rather than only anterior ones).

The third week, Alan targeted /ts/ again. He was not able to target final /ps/ or /ks/, but he could target plurals as a whole, using /s/ rather than postvocalic /z/.

The /s/-clusters which were targeted singly during Cycle One were grouped, two each week. Probing for *It's a* --- phrases revealed that he was not yet ready for them. Word-initial /s/ and word-initial /f/ were targeted during the seventh and eighth weeks. Prevocalic liquids were introduced during the last two weeks of Cycle Two.

When Alan returned for summer school, he was consistently producing final /k/ and was stimulable for initial velars, which he targeted for two weeks. "Easy" words were presented the first week; harder words were targeted the second.

The focus of the remaining four weeks were liquids and liquid clusters. It was perhaps premature for Alan to target /l/-clusters and /r/-clusters during that cycle. We probably should have presented another review of /s/-clusters.

Alan was put on a bi-weekly program in the fall semester, attending once every two weeks. He was still attending the special education cooperative, but he was participating in first grade instructional activities. Stridency and consonant clusters were the focus for Cycle Four. The clusters, /sp/, /st/, /sm/, and /sn/, were presented together during the first week. He was able to target /sk/ the next session and /sl/ in the following lesson. He was finally ready for *It's a* --- phrases, and they were employed for the next two times. During the last session, /r/-clusters were targeted.

Alan came to the university clinic every third week during the spring semester. The first two lessions were "two-pronged," with separate targets for each half. He targeted the palatal affricate /tʃ/ and difficult postvocalic /s/-clusters both sessions. The third lesson was focused on final /ɚ/. Consonant clusters were targeted during the last two weeks.

Alan's phonological posttest results at age 7;5 are shown in Appendix C. He was dismissed from the Phonology Program at the end of the spring semester, having participated for five cycles during a period of 18 months. His speech was not without error, but he was quite intelligible. Furthermore, he was becoming an excellent first grade reader. The following fall semester, he entered a regular second grade classroom in his local community and reportedly was achieving at a high level.

BOBBY (3;6)

Bobby entered the Phonology Program with Level 0 phonological patterns. He produced some glides and nasals. His expressive language consisted mainly of monosyllables and an elaborate gestural system. Receptive language measures indicated that Bobby's receptive language was above average. He had a history of otitis media, but no other significant etiological factors were identified.

Results obtained from Bobby's phonological pretest evaluation (See Appendix C) placed him in the Profound category. He needed to develop both prevocalic and postvocalic obstruent singletons, clusters, the ability to produce more than one syllable, and of course, stridents, velars, liquids, and consonant clusters.

He began by targeting final voiceless stops. Final /p/ was the easiest to elicit. Final /k/ was next easiest, and it was targeted the second week.

"Syllableness" was targeted the following week. Spondee words such as *cowboy* and *baseball*, were used as target words. The next week combinations such as *cowboy hat*, *baseball bat*, and *ice cream cone* were presented. Production of appropriate consonants was not a concern. The goal was to have Bobby produce the appropriate number of syllables. He experienced considerable success while targeting "syllableness." Furthermore, he began putting two and three words together in his spontaneous utterances.

The next target was CVC syllables. Bobby could produce a few final consonants, and a few initial consonants, but he experienced great difficulty producing both beginning and ending consonants in the same word. Therefore, words such as *pipe, pup*, and *pop*, were used to help him realize that there could be beginning and ending sounds in the same word.

Final /t/ and then final /ts/ were targeted the next two weeks. The primary goals were to facilitate final consonants and to elicit some stridency. Bobby was given opportunity to discriminate among minimal contrasts, such as *me, meat, meats*, and *bow, boat, boats*. The concept of "pluralness" was also incorporated in these.

The /ts/ target served to introduce stridency. The next strident target which Bobby was able to produce was /sm/. Liquids were introduced the last two weeks of Bobby's first cycle: initial /l/ and final /ɚ/.

Bobby participated in a group program with other four-year-olds during the summer session. The first week, all of the children targeted "pluralness." Each child received approximately 15 minutes of individual time, during which a couple of minutes of slightly amplified auditory bombardment for the week's target was provided. Also productions were monitored more carefully during this time. The other four weeks of summer session were spent on initial /s/-clusters: /sp/, /st/, /sm/, /sn/.

Bobby returned in the fall semester and targeted stridency, liquids, and consonant clusters. He was dismissed from the Phonology Program at the end of the fall semester. (See Appendix C for posttest results.) During the following spring semester, he participated in an itinerant speech-language program in his local school district. He received programming for syntax and also for /r/. Bobby returned to the university clinic during the summer for re-evaluation. (Results obtained are shown in Appendix C.) He entered kindergarten the following year and reportedly excelled in pre-reading activities.

BARRY (8;9)

Barry attended the Phonology Program for one summer only and received something of a "crash" program. His home was approximately 180 miles from the clinic. The family travelled once a week for five weeks to bring him. Barry had already had five years of speech programming, but still had a great deal of difficulty being understood.

The results obtained from Barry's phonological pretest evaluation (shown in Appendix C) placed him in the Severe category for his age. His major deficiency was consonant clusters. He could produce singleton obstruents fairly well, but Cluster Reduction decreased his intelligibility greatly, particularly in continuous speech. He also experienced a great deal of difficulty with liquids and glides, particularly /r/ and /j/. His scores for Stridency Deletion and Velar Deviations were mostly related to his problem with consonant clusters.

During the first week that Barry attended, four initial /s/-clusters were targeted (/sp, st, sk, sm/). The combinations of /sn/, /sl/, and /sw/ were particularly difficult for him, but he could cope with the other four /s/-clusters at the same time. The next week, the *It's a ---*

carrier phrase was incorporated with his /s/-cluster words.

The third week, Barry targeted prevocalic /r/. At the same time, /j/ was stimulated. However, he was not able to produce an acceptable /j/ until his last week.

The fourth week, Barry targeted /l/ in clusters and in the medial position. He already produced initial /l/ acceptably. Several minutes of the session were spent in trying to elicit /j/.

Barry's last lesson targeted "difficult" /s/-clusters, including medial and final /st/ and /sk/. Also, he succeeded in producing /j/ and was given a few /j/ words to practice.

Needless to say, five weeks was not enough time. Nonetheless, the focus on clusters and the systematic approach of teaching him to replace his major deficient patterns resulted in some gains. Liquids were more facile. There were fewer occurrences of cluster reduction, and he was finally able to produce /j/. Barry's phonological posttest results are shown in Appendix C.

Table 8 – Remediation Cycles for Six Clients*

Jerry

CYCLE ONE**
Prevoc. Velars
/k/ⁱ
Stridency
/sp/
/st/
/f/ⁱ
Liquids
/l/ⁱ
/r/ⁱ

CYCLE TWO
Prevoc. Velars
/k/ⁱ, /g/ⁱ
Stridency
/sp/, /st/
/sm/
/sn/
/sk/
It's a non-/s/
It's a /s/
/tʃ/ᶠ
/f/ᶠ
/f/ⁱ
Liquids
/l/ⁱ
/r/ⁱ

Danny

CYCLE ONE
Postvoc. Velars
/k/ᶠ
Stridency
/ps/
/ts/
/sk/
Liquids
/sp/
/r/ⁱ

CYCLE TWO
Stridency
Plurals
/sk/, /sp/
/st/
/sm/, /sn/
It's a non-/s/
It's a /s/
/s/ⁱ
/f/ⁱ
/tʃ/ⁱ
Liquids
/l/ⁱ
/r/ clus

Tim

CYCLE ONE
Prevoc. Sing. Obs.
/p/ⁱ
/t/ⁱ
/f/ⁱ
/s/ⁱ
/tʃ/ⁱ
/ʃ/ⁱ

CYCLE TWO
Velars
/k/ᶠ
/g/ⁱ
Prevoc. Sing. Obs.
/p/ⁱ, /t/ⁱ
/f/ⁱ, /s/ⁱ
/tʃ/ⁱ, /ʃ/ⁱ
Stridency
/ps/
/ts/
Plurals
/s/ᶠ
/f/ᶠ
/sm/
/sn/

Alan

CYCLE ONE
Postvoc. Sing. Obs.
/p/ᶠ
/t/ᶠ
Velars
/k/ᶠ
Stridency; Clus.
/ts/ᶠ
/st/ⁱ
/sp/ⁱ
/sm/ⁱ
/sn/ⁱ

CYCLE TWO
Velars
/k/ᶠ
Backness
/h/ⁱ
Stridency; Clus.
/ts/ᶠ
Plurals
/sp/, /st/
/sm/, /sn/
/s/ⁱ
/f/ⁱ
Liquids
/l/ⁱ
/r/ⁱ

Bobby

CYCLE ONE
Postvoc. Sing. Obs.
/p/ᶠ
/k/ᶠ
Syllableness
2-Syllables
3-Syllables
CVC
Postvoc. Sing. Obs.
/t/ᶠ
Stridency; Clus.
/ts/ᶠ
/sm/
Liquids
/l/ⁱ
/ɚ/ᶠ

CYCLE TWO
Stridency
Plurals
/sp/
/st/
/sm/
/sn/

Barry

CYCLE ONE
Stridency; Clus.
/sp/, /st/, /sm/, /sk/
It's a (/s/)
Liquids
/r/ⁱ
/l/-clus.
Stridency; Clus.
Difficult /s/-clus.

CYCLE THREE
Clusters
/l/-clus.
/r/-clus.
3-C clus.

Deaff. vs. Aff.
/tʃ/ — /ʃ/
Liquids
/ɝ/ᶠ

CYCLE THREE
Miscellaneous
/j/; Cᴹ
/st/ᴹ, /st/ᶠ
/l/-clus.
/n/ᶠ, /m/ᶠ; /g/ᴵ-/k/ᴵ

CYCLE THREE
Prevoc. Sing. Obs.
/p, t, f, s, tʃ, ʃ/ᴵ
/g/ᴵ
/k/ᴵ
Stridency
/sp/ᴵ
/st/ᴵ
/ps/ᶠ, /ts/ᶠ
Plurals
It's a (non-/s/)
It's a (/s/)
Liquids
/l/ᴵ
/r/ᴵ

CYCLE FOUR
Stridency
/st/ᴵ
/sk/ᶠ
/ks/ᶠ
/sk/ᴵ
Liquids
/l/-clus.
/r/-clus.

CYCLE THREE
Velars
/k/ᴵ
/k/ᴵ; /g/ᴵ
Liquids
/l/ᴵ
/l/-clus.
/r/-clus.

CYCLE FOUR
Stridency; Clus.
/sp/, /st/, /sm/, /sn/
/sk/
/sl/
It's a (non-/s/)
It's a /s/
Liquids
/r/-clus.

CYCLE FIVE
Affrication; Stridency
/tʃ/ᶠ, /st/ᶠ
/tʃ/ᶠ, /sk/ᶠ
Liquids
/ɝ/
/r/-clus.
3-C clus.

CYCLE THREE
Stridency
plurals
/sp/, /st/
/sm/, /sn/
/sk/
It's a (non-/s/)
It's a (/s/)
Liquids
/l/ᴵ
/r/ᴵ
/l/-clus.
/r/-clus.

* See case study for each client for explanation of individual deficiencies and capabilities.
** In each cycle, the target patterns are identified and the phonemes through which they were targeted are listed on separate lines. Each line on which a phoneme or phonemes are given represents a week of training.

Chapter 7

Adapting the Program to the Public Schools

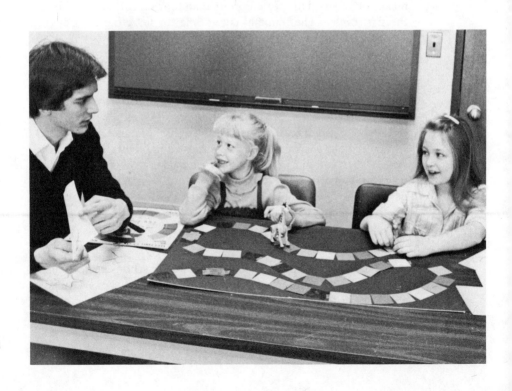

Since our implementation of the approach to phonological remediation described in the previous chapters took place within the setting of a university speech and hearing clinic, the specifics such as session and cycle length represent our adaptation to the requirements of that environment. Such details, of course, are not the essentials of the approach. The remediation principles discussed in Chapter 4 and their resultant effects upon programming described in Chapter 5 are basic, but these elements can be maintained while adjusting to the routine of the setting within which the remediation will take place. Graduates of our program and workshop participants have reported numerous creative adaptations to meet the particular requirements of their professional unit and the needs of their unintelligible clients. Since the setting within which the child with delayed phonological development most commonly receives professional assistance is the public school, this chapter will deal with specific suggestions for adjusting the program to that environment.

TIME TO FOCUS ON A TARGET PHONEME

It has proved to be expedient to target each major pattern by means of no less than two nor more than four specific targets during the first cycle. The minimal clinic time for targeting each of the specific phonemes or phoneme sequences within the pattern is 60 minutes. Thus, if 20 minutes is the session length set by the school, three sessions might be devoted to a given target phoneme before progressing to the next. Suggested time-allotments in a 20-minute clinic session are given in Table 9. If the sessions are 30 minutes, however, two sessions per target would be sufficient. Two 30-minute or three 20-minute sessions per week would thus make it possible to spend only one week per target as we have done. During subsequent cycles, when two or three targets are grouped together for review, the resulting unit would be focused upon for the same 60-minute total period before moving on to a new target within the pattern or to another recycled pattern.

GROUPING OF CLIENTS

The large caseload assigned to most public school professionals may require that children be seen in small groups whenever this is appropriate for the individual child's needs. Our experience has shown that children who are functioning at Level 0 or using Level I patterns need individual sessions. Those who are targeting Level II

**Table 9 — *Sample Time Schedule for 20-minute Public School
Session***

1:00	Review last session's picture-word cards
1:02	Auditory bombardment of words for this session's target
1:04	Child draws 2 to 3 picture cards (Clinician writes word on card)
1:08	Activity No. 1 (e.g., maze)
1:12	Activity No. 2 (e.g., concentration; reading for older children)
1:17	Probing to determine next session's target
1:18	Repeat auditory bombardment
1:20	Dismissal (Child takes cards and word list for practice.)

patterns usually progress fairly well in a group situation. Activities
involving /s/-clusters are particularly well-suited for group participation, even when the children are targeting different /s/-clusters.
Needless to say, the children in a group must be working toward the
same desired pattern, but individual deficiencies do not need to be
identical.

DAILY REVIEW PROGRAM

After we began incorporating a home program, its usefulness as
described in Chapter 6 was clearly evident. Although it required only
five minutes or less per day for the child to listen to a 15-word list and
to name his week's practice words, the daily reminder served as a
valuable reinforcement for the new image. Consequently, we urge
that a daily program be arranged to accompany public school
training.

Many parents are anxious to cooperate, even if they are unable to
come to school to observe and/or receive instructions. However, in
other instances and for a variety of reasons, parent participation is not
available. Speech-language pathologists we know have used a variety
of improvisations to fill this gap. If there are aides employed by the

school, this task is very appropriate for their role. In some situations, older elementary school pupils in the same building have been contracted to perform this task. Some clinicians have prepared audiotapes and arranged for the child to listen to his word list daily at some listening station in the school. The daily stimulation keeps the auditory image in the forefront of the child's consciousness and its contribution is of sufficient importance to warrant seeking some means for accomplishing it even if only for five days per week rather than for seven.

MEETING PUBLIC LAW 94-142 REQUIREMENTS

The highly individualized nature of this phonological approach satisfies requirements for Public Law 94-142. The rapid intelligibility gains more quickly serve the child's needs and tend to reduce the handicapping effects on academic progress. Furthermore, reducing the total length of remediation time for a client serves the clinician's need for reducing caseload size.

A sample IEP is illustrated in Table 10. The goal of a phonological approach is to increase intelligibility by teaching major phonological patterns. In most schools, administrators accept a statement of objectives such as those shown. The cycles can be written in as the year progresses. Posttest scores satisfy the need for accountability measures.

OTHER CONSIDERATIONS

The Severity Intervals proposed in Chapter 3 may be especially useful to the public school speech-language pathologist. When objective measures are required to select caseloads, define priority clients, and determine time allotments, the suggested Composite Phonological Deviancy Scores may be a realistic basis for comparison of client needs.

In many ways, the public school setting provides an opportunity for more comprehensive programming. Self-contained communicative disorders classrooms, in particular, may serve as an excellent means for combining language, phonology, and remedial education goals.

Table 10 —*Sample IEP*

Goal: To increase intelligibility by facilitating emergence of the following phonological patterns:

		Criterion*	When Achieved
Final consonants			
Velars			
Stridency			
Consonant clusters			
Liquids			

Behavioral Objectives:

1. _____ will listen to approximately
   (name)
   15 target pattern words.

2. _____ will draw 2-to-5 pictures of target words on 5"-x-8" index cards.

3. _____ will produce the target by naming the picture cards while participating in 2-to-5 experiential play activities.

4. _____ will again listen to target pattern words.

Cycles:

(To be filled in as program progresses.)

*The criterion may be specified as 100% for any child who is capable of the tasks.

REFERENCES

Bankson, N.W., & Bernthal, J.E. A comparison of phonological processes identified through word and sentence imitation tasks of the PPA. *Language, Speech, and Hearing Services in Schools,* 1982, *13*, 96-99.

Blache, S.E., & Parsons, C.L. A linguistic approach to distinctive feature training. *Language, Speech, and Hearing Services in Schools,* 1980, *11*, 203-207.

Blache, S.E., Parsons, C.L., & Humphreys, J.M. A minimal word-pair model for teaching the linguistic significance of distinctive feature properties. *Journal of Speech and Hearing Disorders,* 1981, *46*, 291-296.

Chomsky, N., & Halle, M. *The sound pattern of English.* New York: Harper and Row, 1968.

Clifton, L.B., & Elliott, L.L. CV identification thresholds for speech/language/learning-disordered listeners. *Journal of the Acoustical Society of America,* 1982, *71*, S57.

Compton, A.J. Generative studies in children's phonological disorders. *Journal of Speech and Hearing Disorders,* 1970, *35*, 315-339.

Compton, A.J. Generative studies of children's phonological disorders: a strategy of therapy. In S. Singh (Ed.), *Measurement procedures in speech, hearing, and language.* Baltimore: University Park Press, 1975.

Compton, A.J. Studies of early child phonology. San Francisco: Institute of Child Language and Phonology, unpublished report, 1977.

Compton, A.J., & Hutton, J.S. *The Compton-Hutton phonological assessment.* San Francisco: Carousel House, 1978.

Costello, J., & Onstine, J.M. The modification of multiple articulation errors based on distinctive feature theory. *Journal of Speech and Hearing Disorders*, 1976, *41*, 199-215.

Dunn, C., & Barron, C. A treatment program for disordered phonology: Phonetic and linguistic considerations. *Language, Speech, and Hearing Services in Schools*, 1982, *13*, 100-109.

Dyson, A.M.T. *Strategies toward the suppression of five phonological simplification processes by two-year-olds,* Unpublished doctoral dissertation, University of Illinois, 1979.

Edwards, M.L. *Patterns and processes in fricative acquisition: Longitudinal evidence from six English-learning children.* Doctoral dissertation, Stanford University, 1978.

Edwards, M.L., & Bernhardt, B. *Phonological analyses of the speech of four children with language disorders.* Unpublished manuscript. Stanford University, 1973.

Elliott, L.L., & Katz, D. *The Northwestern University-children's perception of speech test* (NU-CHIPS). St. Louis: Auditec, 1980.

Elliott, L. L., Longinotti, C., Clifton, L., & Meyer, D. Detection and identification thresholds for consonant-vowel syllables. *Perception and Psychophysics*, 1981, *30*, 411-416.

Fairbanks, G. Systematic research in experimental phonetics: 1. A theory of the speech mechanism as a servosystem. *Journal of Speech and Hearing Disorders*, 1954, *19*, 133-139.

Gallagher, T., & Shriner, T. Articulatory inconsistencies in the speech of normal development. *Journal of Speech and Hearing Research*, 1975, *18*, 168-175. (a)

Gallagher, T., & Shriner, T. Contextual variables related to inconsistent /s/ and /z/ production. *Journal of Speech and Hearing Research*, 1975, *18*, 623-633. (b)

Hodson, B.W. *The Assessment of phonological processes.* Danville, Il.: Interstate Printers and Publishers, 1980.

Hodson, B.W. Evaluation and remediation of phonological disorders. *Communicative Disorders: An Audio Journal for Continuing Education,* 1981, *6* (4).

Hodson, B.W., Chin, L., Redmond, B., & Simpson, R. Phonological evaluation and remediation of speech deviations of a child with a repaired cleft palate: A case study. *Journal of Speech and Hearing Disorders,* in press.

Hodson, B.W., & Paden, E.P. Phonological processes which characterize unintelligible and intelligible speech in early childhood. *Journal of Speech and Hearing Disorders,* 1981, *46,* 369-373.

Ingram, D. *Phonological disability in children.* New York: Elsevier, 1976.

Ingram, D. *Procedures for the phonological analysis of children's language.* Baltimore: University Park Press, 1981.

Jakobson, R., Fant, C.M., & Halle, M. *Preliminaries to speech analysis.* Cambridge, Mass.: M.I.T. Press, 1952.

Kent, R.D. Contextual facilitation of correct sound production. *Language, Speech, and Hearing Services in Schools,* 1982, *13,* 66-76.

McReynolds, L.V., & Bennett, S. Distinctive feature generalization in articulation training. *Journal of Speech and Hearing Disorders,* 1972, *37,* 462-470.

McReynolds, L.V., & Huston, K. A distinctive feature analysis of children's misarticulations. *Journal of Speech and Hearing Disorders,* 1971, *36,* 155-166.

Moss, S.A. A comparison of phonological assessment results based on a conversational speech sample versus an elicited word list. Unpublished study, University of Illinois, 1982.

Ruder, K.F., & Bunce, B.H. Articulation therapy using distinctive feature analysis to structure the training program: Two case studies. *Journal of Speech and Hearing Disorders*, 1981, *46*, 59-65.

Shriberg, L.D. Developmental phonological disorders. In T.J. Hixon, L.D. Shriberg & J.H. Saxman (Eds.), *Introduction to communication disorders,* Englewood Cliffs, N.J.: Prentice-Hall, 1980.

Shriberg, L.D., & Kwiatkowski, J. *Natural process analysis.* New York: John Wiley and Sons, 1980.

Singh, S. *Distinctive features: Theory and validation.* Baltimore: University Park Press, 1976.

Smith, N.V. *The acquisition of phonology.* London: Cambridge University Press, 1973.

Stampe, D. The acquisition of phonetic representation. *Papers from the Fifth Regional Meeting of the Chicago Linguistic Society,* 1969, 443-454.

Swisher, W.E. An investigation of physiologically and acoustically facilitating phonetic environments on the production and perception of defective speech sounds. Doctoral dissertation. University of Wisconsin, 1973.

Templin, M.C. *Certain language skills in children.* Minneapolis: University of Minnesota Press, 1957.

Van Riper, C. *Speech correction: Principles and methods.* New York: Prentice-Hall, 1939.

Weiner, F. *Phonological process analysis.* Baltimore: University Park Press, 1979.

Weiner, F. Treatment of phonological disability using the method of meaningful minimal contrast: Two case studies. *Journal of Speech and Hearing Disorders.* 1981, *46,* 97-103.

Weiner, F., & Bankson, N. Teaching features. *Language, Speech, and Hearing Services in Schools,* 1978, *9,* 24-28.

Weismer, G., Dinnsen, D., & Elbert, M. A study of the voicing distinction associated with omitted word-final stops. *Journal of Speech and Hearing Disorders,* 1981, *46,* 320-328.

Young, E., & Hawk, S. *Moto-kinesthetic speech training.* Palo Alto: Stanford University Press, 1955.

GLOSSARY

Affricates. Consonants for which there is a complete stoppage of the outgoing breath stream followed by a relatively slow, turbulent release: /tʃ, dʒ/.

Alveolars. Consonants produced by placing the tongue on or close to the alveolar ridge (the gum ridge just behind the upper teeth): /t, d, n, l, s, z/.

Apicalization. Production of a non-apical sound with the tip of the tongue raised.

Auditory cue. Any use of the sense of hearing for drawing attention to a phonemic characteristic.

Auditory training unit. An electronic device that allows words spoken into a microphone to be amplified before being delivered to earphones.

Backing. Replacing an anterior consonant with one which is produced in the velar or glottal region.

Bilabials. Consonants produced by bringing the lips together: /p, b, m, w/.

Coalescence. Replacement of two adjacent phonemes by a single sound which is neither of the originals, but retains features of both.

Composite Phonological Deviancy Score. A number which reflects the mean strength of a child's basic deficient patterns, plus any additional critical patterns he may be using, as well as an adjustment which adds points for 4, 5, 6, 7-and-older ages which helps provide priority ratings.

Consonant cluster. Two or more consecutive consonants in the same syllable.

Consonant singleton. A single consonant which occurs before or after a vowel in a syllable.

Cycle. A consecutive time period of about two to three months during which a group of phonological patterns is sequentially targeted, usually for two to four weeks per pattern.

Dentalization. Production of an alveolar consonant with the tongue in a more forward position (i.e., against or between the teeth).

Devoicing. Deletion of voicing from a typically voiced sound.

Diminutive. Addition of /i/ to a word; frequently observed in the speech of normally-developing 2-year-olds.

Distinctive feature. A characteristic of a phoneme which is essential to its identity as distinct from other phonemes.

Epenthesis. Insertion of an additional phone somewhere in a word.

Foil word. A word that serves to contrast a deficient pattern with the desired form.

Fricatives. Consonants for which the articulators are loosely approximated so that turbulence is created in the outgoing breath stream: /f, v, s, z, ʃ, ʒ, θ, ð, h/.

Fronting. Replacing a consonant with sound produced farther forward in the oral cavity.

Glides. Prevocalic consonants characterized by a rapid movement of the articulators from a high front or back tongue arch to the vowel that follows: /w, j/.

Gliding. Replacing a phoneme from another consonant class with a glide; most often, replacing a liquid with a glide.

Glottal replacement. Replacing a consonant with a glottal stop.

Glottal stop. A sound produced by stopping the air flow at the vocal folds, with or without a subsequent plosive release: /ʔ/.

Idiosyncratic rule. An uncommon deficient phonological pattern.

Interdentals. Consonants produced by placing the tongue between the front teeth: /θ, ð/.

Intervocalic. The sequential position in a word of a consonant between vowels.

Kinesthetic. The sense of the position or movement of (articulatory) structures by means of the end-organs of muscles within those structures.

Labials. Consonants in which the lips are used to block or constrict the outgoing breath stream: /p, b, m, w, f, v/.

Labiodentals. Consonants produced by touching the lower lip to the upper teeth: /f, v/.

Lateralization. Production of a typically non-lateral phoneme with one or both sides of the tongue lowered so that air escapes to the side.

Liquids. Consonants for which the articulators make only partial, frictionless approximation: /r, l/.

Metathesis. Reversal of sequential position of two sounds or syllables in an utterance, often, but not always, within the same word.

Migration. Transfer of sound to another position in the utterance, usually within the same word.

Minimal pairs. Two words which are alike in all but one phoneme.

Nasalization. Production of a typically non-nasal sound with nasal emission.

Nasals. Consonants produced by blocking the oral cavity and emitting the sound through the nose: /m, n, ŋ/.

Natural phonology. A theory proposed by Stampe (1969) which hypothesizes that children have an innate set of processes for simplifying the adult target words to a level which they are capable of producing, and which suggests that children must learn to suppress these processes to acquire adult speech.

Natural process. A sound change which results in a less complex structure at the surface level and which occurs frequently in natural languages of the world.

Neutralization. Lack of differentiation between vowels so that several are reduced to the same phoneme.

Obstruents. Consonants which are not spontaneously voiced (i.e., have voiceless cognates): fricatives, stops, affricates.

Palatals. Consonants for which the tongue is raised toward the hard palate: /ʃ, ʒ, tʃ, dʒ, j, r/.

Pharyngealization. Production of a consonant with constriction in the pharyngeal area.

Phone. A single speech sound produced by a speaker in one utterance.

Phoneme. A group of sounds which are similar acoustically and in articulatory gesture and comprise the smallest segment of meaningful utterance that is distinguished in contrast with other such segments.

Phonological pattern. The standard adult speech patterns of a linguistic community including sound classes, syllable shapes, and syllable sequences.

Phonological process or deficient pattern. A regularly occurring deviation from standard adult speech patterns; may occur across a class of sounds, a syllable shape, or syllable sequence.

Phonological rule. The specification of a particular change regularly observed in oral language and the exact conditions under which it occurs.

Phonology. The sound structure of language, characterized by a finite set of phonemes and specific arrangements in which they can be combined into syllables.

Postvocalic. The sequential position in a syllable following the vowel.

Prevocalic. The sequential position in a syllable preceding the vowel.

Probing. Stimulating by means of one or two carefully selected words in order to determine whether a child is capable of producing a desired sound or sequence.

Reduplication. Repetition of the same syllable or sound in place of two or more phonemically different units.

Servosystem. A mechanism in which output is compared to intent so that its characteristics can be judged and corrected.

Severity intervals. Groupings of Composite Phonological Deviancy Scores as a means of indicating relative needs for intervention.

Sibilants. Consonants which can be described as "hissing" sounds: /s, z, ʃ, ʒ, tʃ, dʒ/.

Sonorants. Consonants in which the flow of air is relatively unobstructed, and which are characterized by vowel-like acoustic energy: nasals, liquids and glides. Vowels are also sonorants.

Stopping. Replacing any continuant consonant with a stop.

Stops. Consonants for which there is a complete stoppage of the outgoing breath stream, usually followed by an abrupt release: /p, b, t, d, k, g/.

Stridency deletion. Omission of the strident feature by substitution of a non-strident sound, or by omitting the phoneme altogether.

Stridents. Consonants characterized by considerable noisy turbulence caused by forceful air flow striking the back of the teeth: /f, v, s, z, ∫, ʒ, t∫, dʒ/.

Syllabic. A consonant which fulfills the vowel function in a syllable.

Syllableness. Production of the target number of syllable units within a word without concern for their phonemic correctness.

Tactual cue. Use of the sense of touch for drawing attention to a phonemic characteristic.

Target pattern. The adult sound class, syllable shape or syllable sequence which the child needs to acquire.

Target phoneme. The phoneme (or combination of phonemes) within a pattern which is being facilitated by auditory stimulation and production practice.

Velarization. Production of a non-velar consonant with constriction in the velar area.

Velars. Consonants produced by arching the back of the tongue to make contact with the soft palate (velum): /k, g, ŋ/.

Visual cue. Any visual means for drawing attention to a phonemic characteristic.

Voicing. Addition of voicing to a typically voiceless sound.

Vowelization. Replacing a postvocalic or syllabic liquid with a vowel, usually /ʊ, ɔ, o, ʌ, ə/.

APPENDIX A

Cross-Listing of Consonant
Sound Classifications

	/p/	/b/	/t/	/d/	/k/	/g/	/f/	/v/	/θ/	/ð/	/s/	/z/	/ʃ/	/ʒ/	/tʃ/	/dʒ/	/m/	/n/	/ŋ/	/r/	/l/	/w/	/j/	/h/
Obstruents	✓	✓	✓	✓	✓	✓	✓	✓	✓	✓	✓	✓	✓	✓	✓	✓								✓
Sonorants																	✓	✓	✓	✓	✓	✓	✓	
Stops	✓	✓	✓	✓	✓	✓																		
Fricatives							✓	✓	✓	✓	✓	✓	✓	✓										✓
Affricates															✓	✓								
Liquids																				✓	✓			
Nasals																	✓	✓	✓					
Glides																						✓	✓	
Stridents							✓	✓			✓	✓	✓	✓	✓	✓								
Sibilants											✓	✓	✓	✓	✓	✓								
Labials	✓	✓					✓	✓									✓					✓		
Interdentals									✓	✓														
Alveolars			✓	✓							✓	✓						✓		✓	✓			
Palatals													✓	✓	✓	✓				✓			✓	
Velars					✓	✓													✓			✓		
Glottals																								✓
Voiced		✓		✓		✓		✓		✓		✓		✓		✓	✓	✓	✓	✓	✓	✓	✓	
Voiceless	✓		✓		✓		✓		✓		✓		✓		✓									✓

APPENDIX B

Answers to Exercises

Answers to Exercise 1 — Identifying Phonological Processes.

Productions	Omissions Only		Omissions or Substitutions			Other Sonorants		Assimilations	Other
	Cluster Reduction	Singleton Obstruents	Stridency Deletion	Velar Deviations	Liquid Deviations	Nasals	Glides		
soap →									
/toʊ/		/s/ /p/ ✓	/s/ ✓						Stopping
/haʊ/		✓	✓						Backing
/boʊpl/			✓					Labial	Stopping, Prevocal. Voice
watch →									
/wat/		/g/	/g/ ✓				/w/		Deaffrication, Depalataliz.
/a/		✓	✓				✓		
/ha?/		?	✓				✓		Backing, Glottal Replac
string →									
/twi/	/str/ ✓		/s/ ✓	/ŋ/	/r/				Gliding
/nin/	✓ ✓		✓	✓	✓	/ŋ/ ✓		Nasal	Fronting
/kwiŋ/	✓		✓	✓	✓			Velar ~ Backing	Gliding, Backing
screw-driver →									
/tu daɪ bʌ/	/skr/ /dr/ /v/ ✓ ✓		/s/ /v/ ✓	/k/ ✓	/r/ /r/ /ə/ ✓			Alveolar	Stopping, Vowelization
/kwʊ gaɪ ə/	✓		✓	✓	✓			Velar ~ Backing	Fronting, Gliding
/pu bwaɪ/	✓ ✓		✓	✓	✓			Labial	Syllable Reduc., Fronting, Gliding

~ Indicates that either one or the other of the patterns shown is occurring. More examples of the child's productions would need to be evaluated in order to determine which pattern should be tallied.

Answers to Exercise 2 — Identifying Phonological Systems.

Target	A (5;11)	J (5;7)	D (5;6)	T (5;0)
/fɹæk/	/bʌ/	/pɔwk/	/hou/	/ɔɪʔ/
/nouz/	/mou/	/nous/	/nou/	/ɹoud/
/glʌv/	/bʌ/	/dʌb/	/kʌ/	/dʌb̥/
/strɪŋ/	/nɪ/	/tɪŋ/	/hɪm/	/ɪn/
/kreɪ ənz/	/na/	/teɪ ən/	/keɪ am/	/eɪ ənt/
/aɪs kjubz/	/aɪ tʲu/	/aɪ tʌps/	/aɪ kjup/	/aɪ ʊd/
/skru draɪ vɚ/	/tu daɪ wu/	/tu daɪ bu/	/ku kaw ɚ/	/u daɪ bu/
/tɛ lə vɪ ʒən/	/bɛ ə tɪ jə/	/tɛ bə bɪ bən/	/tɛ ə bɪ wəm/	/ɛl ə bɪ dɛn/
/θʌm/	/pʌm/	/pʌm/	/hʌm/	/ʌm/

List below each process which is used at least twice by that child.

	A (5;11)	J (5;7)	D (5;6)	T (5;0)
	Cluster Reduction and Postvocalic Cluster Deletion	Cluster Reduction	Cluster Reduction	Cluster Reduction and Prevocalic Cluster Deletion
	Liquid Deviation	Liquid Deviation	Liquid Deviation (some good /ɚ/)	Liquid Deviation
	Stridency Deletion	Stridency Deletion (some good final /s/	Stridency Deletion	Stridency Deletion
	Final Consonant Deletion	—	Some Final Consonant Deletion	Prevocalic Voiceless Obstruent Deletion
	Velar Deviation	Prevocalic Velar Fronting	Postvocalic Velar Deviation	Velar Deviation
	Glide Syllables	Stopping	Prevocalic Backing	Glottal Replacement
	Nasal Assimilation	Reduplication	Final Nasal → /m/	Stopping
	Stopping	Postvocalic Devoicing	Prevocalic Devoicing	Postvocalic Devoicing

Who said /hʌm/ /hʌm/ /ʌm/ /pʌm/ for the target /θʌm/? (Fill in the predicted production of thumb for each child.)

Answers to Exercise 3 — *Determining Composite Phonological Deviancy Scores and Severity Intervals*

Basic Deficient Patterns (with possible numbers of occurrences)	A(5;11)	J(5;7)	D(5;6)	T(5;0)
	Percentage of Occurrence			
Syllable Reduction (21)	10	0	0	5
Cluster Reduction (35)	106*	86	97	131*
Obstruent Singleton Omission				
Prevocalic (38)	8	3	11	42
Postvocalic (30)	97	10	83	37
Stridency Deletion (44)	100	59	91	100
Velar Deviation (24)	100	54	46	100
Liquid Deviation				
/l/ (13)	92	100	85	92
/r, ɚ/ (26)	100	100	58	100
Nasal Deviation (19)	53	0	0	5
Glide Deviation (10)	60	30	10	50
Total	736	442	481	662
Average	74	44	48	66

Other Level I and II Patterns	A(5;11)	J(5;7)	D(5;6)	T(5;0)
	Frequency of Occurrence			
Vowel Deviation	5 1		5 1	1
Prevocalic Voicing	14 4			6 2
Prevocalic Devoicing			5 1	
Glottal Replacement	1		2	8 2
Backing		3 1	12 4	
Stopping	14 4	19 6	5 1	19 6
Coalescence			1	
Epenthesis		5 1	1	1
Metathesis	1	1	1	
Assimiliation				
Nasal	6 2			
Velar			3 1	
Labial	5 1	6 2	1	3 1
Idiosyncratic Patterns				
Glide Syllable	13 4		4 1	
Final /n, ŋ/→/m/			11 3	
Nasal Addition/Replacement				6 2
Total Additional Pattern Points	16	10	12	13

	A(5;11)	J(5;7)	D(5;6)	T(5;0)
Percentage Average	74	44	48	66
Additional Pattern Points	16	10	12	13
Age Points for 5-year-olds	10	10	10	10
Total	100	64	70	89
Severity Intervals	High Profound	Severe	Severe	Profound

---

* Percentages above 100 reflect Cluster Deletion as well as Cluster Reduction, since one instance of cluster reduction is tallied for each segment (sound) that is missing.

APPENDIX C

**Pre- and Posttest
Responses and Phonological
Analysis Scores of Six Clients**

JERRY: 5;7, 6;3

JERRY: 5;7, 6;3

Target	Pretest	Posttest
airplane	'eʊdeɪn	'eʊpweɪn
basket	'bæt̪ɪt̪	'baskɪt
bed	bɛd	bɛd
candle	'tænʊ	'kændʊ
chair	tɛʊ	ʃɛʊ
cowboy hat	'taʊbɔɪˌhæt	'kaʊbɔɪˌhæt
crayons	'teɪən	'kreɪənz̥
three	ti	fwi
black	dæk	blæk
green	din	grin
yellow	'dɛwoʊ	'lɛwoʊ
doll	da:	da:
feather	'pɛhʊ	'fɛðu

Target	Pretest	Posttest
page	peɪts	peɪʒ
quarter	'toʊtʊ	'kwɔʊtʊ
rouge	wʊs	wʊtʃ
rug	wʌg̥	rʌg
Santa Claus	'sænhiˌtɔwi	'sæntəˌkwɔz
skrewdriver	'tuˌdaɪbʊ	'skruˌdraɪvu
shoe	su	ʃu
sled	dɛd	slɛd
smooth	mʌp	smʌv
snake	neɪk	sneɪk
soap	s:oup	soup
spoon	pʌn	spʌn
spring	θɪŋ	spwɪŋ

Word		
fish	pɪʃ	fɪʃ
flower	'sauwu	'flauwu
fork	pɔuk	fɔuk
glasses	dæhɪ	'glæsɪz̥
glove	dʌb̥	glʌv
gun	dʌn	gʌn
hanger	'hæŋu	'hæŋʊ
horse	'housi	hous
ice cubes	'aɪtubz̥	'aɪskjubz
jumprope	'zʌmp,boup	'zʌmp,woup
leaf	dip	lif
mask	mæks	mæsk
mouth	maup	mauf
music box	'mjuzɪk,bɒks	'mjuzɪk,bɒks
nose	nouz̥	nouz
squirrel	tuwə	skwu:
star	tawə	stau
string	tɪŋ	stwɪŋ
sweater	'wetu	'swetu
television	'tɛbə,bɪbən	'tɛlə,vɪʒən
that	dæt	læt
thumb	pʌm	fʌm
toothbrush	'tu,bʌs	'tuf,bwʌʃ
truck	sʌk	ʃrʌk
tub	tʌb̥	tʌb̥
vase	beɪs	veɪs
watch	wats	watʃ
yoyo	'jou wjou	'jou jou
zipper	'zɪpu	'zɪpu

JERRY

Basic Patterns	Pretest (5;7)	Posttest (6;3)
Syllable Reduction	0%	0%
Cluster Reduction	86	0
Prevocalic Singleton Obstruent Omission	3	0
Postvocalic Singleton Obstruent Omission	10	0
Stridency Deletion	59	0
Velar Deviation	54	0
/l/ Deviation	100	38
/r, ɝ/ Deviation	100	77
Nasal Deviation	0	0
Glide Deviation	30	0
Total	442	115
Average	44.2=44	11.5=12
Vowel Deviation	0 times	0 times
Prevocalic Voicing	0	0
Postvocalic Devoicing	7	4
Glottal Replacement	0	0
Backing	3	0
Stopping	19	0
Affrication	0	1
Deaffrication	2	3
Palatalization	0	1
Depalatalization	9	0
Coalescence	0	0
Epenthesis	5	1
Metathesis	1	1
Assimilation		
Nasal	0	0
Velar	0	0
Labial	6	0
Alveolar	1	1
"th"→ /f, v, s, z/	0	5
Frontal Lisp	0	0
Dentalization of /t, d, n, l/	3	0
Lateralization	0	0
Other		
Diminutive	2	0
Reduplication	1	0

DANNY: 5;6, 6;5, 6;11

DANNY: 5;6, 6;5, 6;11

Target	Pretest	Posttest	Re-eval.
airplane	ˈɛɔhɛɪm	ˈɛɔpleɪn	ˈɛɔpleɪn
basket	ˈbaʔɪt	ˈbaskɪt	ˈbeskɪt
bed	bɛɔ	bɛd	bed
candle	ˈkæmo	ˈkæno	ˈkændḷ
chair	hɛɔ	tʃɛɔ	tʃɛɔ
cowboy hat	ˈkabo,hæ	ˈkaubɔɪ,hæt	ˈkaubɔɪ,hæt
crayons	ˈkeɪæm	ˈkreɪənz	ˈkreɪənz
three	sɪ	fri	fri
black	bæ	blæk	blæk
green	kɪm	krɪn	grɪn
yellow	ˈlɛwou	ˈjɛlou	ˈjɛlou
doll	daɪ	daː	daɪ
feather	ˈsɛwɔ	ˈfɛvɔ	ˈfɛvɔ
fish	sʲɪ	fɪʃ	fɪʃ

Target	Pretest	Posttest	Re-eval.
page	peɪ	peɪs	peɪdʒ
quarter	ˈkowɔ	ˈkɔɔtɔ̞	ˈkɔɔtɔ
rouge	wu	ruʒ	ruʒ
rug	wʌ	rʌg	rʌg
Santa Claus	ˈkæmi,kɔ	ˈsænwə,klɔz	ˈsænwə,klɔz
skrewdriver	ˈku,kauɔ	ˈsu,graɪvɔ	ˈskrugraɪvɔ
shoe	ʃu	ʃu	ʃu
sled	he	slɛd	slɛd
smooth	mu	smuv	smuʒ
snake	neɪ	sneɪk	sneɪk
soap	houp	soup	soup
spoon	pʌm	spun	spun
spring	pɪm	sprɪŋ	sprɪŋ
squirrel	ksɔ	skwɔl	skwɔl

flower	'sauwɚ	'flauwɚ	'flauwɚ
fork	ho	fouk	fɔɔk
glasses	'kaʔa	'klæhiz̥	'glæsiz
glove	kʌ	klʌv	glʌv
gun	kʌm	kʌm	gʌm
hanger	'hæmɚ	'hæjo	'hæjɚ
horse	ho	hous	hɔɚs
ice cubes	'alkjub	'akjubz̥	'aikjubz
jumprope	dʌm,woup	'dʒʌmpɪroup	'dʒʌmpɪroup
leaf	fʕi	lip	lif
mask	mæt	mæks	mæsk
mouth	mau	mauf	mauθ
music box	'mjuɪ,bak	'muwik,baks	'mjuzik,baks
nose	nou	nouz̥	nouz̥

*pharyngealized

star	taɚ	staɚ	staɚ
string	him	striŋ	striŋ
sweater	'hɛwɚ	'swɛʔɚ	'swɛʔɚ
television	'tɛɚ,biwɚm	'tɛwɚ,biwɚn	'tɛlɚ,viʒɚn
that	dæ	dæt	dæt
thumb	hʌm	fʌm	θʌm
toothbrush	'tu,bʌ	'tu,braʃ	'tu,braʃ
truck	kʌ	trak	trak
tub	hʌb	tʌb	tʌb
vase	beɪ	veɪs	veɪs
watch	wat	watʃ	watʃ
yoyo	'wouwou	'joujou	'joujou
zipper	'tɪɚ	'zɪpɚ	'zɪpɚ

DANNY

Basic Patterns	Pretest (5;6)	Posttest (6;5)	Reevaluation* (6;11)
Syllable Reduction	0%	0%	0%
Cluster Reduction	97	11	6
Prevocalic Singleton Obstruent Omission	11	3	0
Postvocalic Singleton Obstruent Omission	83	7	7
Stridency Deletion	91	14	2
Velar Deviation	46	4	0
/l/ Deviation	85	23	0
/r, ɚ/ Deviation	58	15	0
Nasal Deviation	0	0	0
Glide Deviation	10	30	10
Total	481	107	25
Average	48.1=48	10.7=11	2.5=3
Vowel Deviation	5 times	1 times	0 times
Prevocalic Voicing	0	0	0
Postvocalic Devoicing	1	5	4
Glottal Replacement	2	1	0
Backing	12	2	0
Stopping	5	3	1
Affrication	0	0	0
Deaffrication	3	1	0
Palatalization	0	0	0
Depalatalization	7	2	0
Coalescence	0	0	0
Epenthesis	1	0	0
Metathesis	1	1	0
Assimilation			
Nasal	0	0	0
Velar	3	1	1
Labial	1	1	0
Alveolar	0	0	0
"th"→/f, v, s, z/	1	5	3
Frontal Lisp	0	0	0
Dentalization of /t, d, n, l/	0	0	0
Lateralization	0	0	0
Other			
Postvocalic /n, ŋ/→/m/	11	0	0
Prevocalic devoicing	5	4	0
Glide Syllable	4	3	1

*Danny was available for re-evaluation six months
after his dismissal from the Phonology Program.

TIM: 5;0, 6;1

TIM: 5;0, 6;1

Target	Pretest	Posttest	Target	Pretest	Posttest
airplane	'ɛʊʔeɪn	'ɛɾpweɪn	page	eɪt	peɪdʒ
basket	'bædɛʔ	'bædɪt	quarter	'ʊpɛn	'kwɔɚtɚ
bed	bɛd	bɛd	rouge	wʊʒ̥	rʊʒ
candle	'ændʊ	'kændʊ	rug	wʌg̥	rʌg
chair	ɛʊ	ʃɛʊ	Santa Claus	'ænʔˌʔɔt	'sænəˌklɔz
cowboy hat	'aʊbɔɪˌhæʔ	'kaʊbɔɪˌhæʔ	skrewdriver	'uˌdaɪbʊ	'skuˌdaɪvɚ
crayons	'eɪænʔ	'kɹeɪənz̥	shoe	u	ʃu
three	i	tɹi	sled	ɛd̥	slɛd
black	bæʔ	bwæk	smooth	mʌd̥	smʌv
green	dɪn	gɹɪn	snake	neɪʔ	sneɪk
yellow	'djɛdoʊ	jɛloʊ	soap	oʊp	soʊp
doll	nɑː	dɑl	spoon	bʊn	spʊn
feather	'ɛdɚ	fɛdɚ	spring	mbɪn	spɹɪŋ

word	pretest	posttest
fish	ɪt	fɪʃ
flower	ˈauwu	ˈflauwu
fork	ɔɪʔ	fɔɔk
glasses	ˈdæʌt	ˈglæʔɪz
glove	dʌb̥	glʌv
gun	dʌn	gʌn
hanger	ˈhaɪʔdu	ˈhaɪjæ
horse	hɔɪt	hɔɔs
ice cubes	ˈaɪud̥	ˈaɪkjubd
jumprope	ˈdʌmʔˌwoup	ˈdʒʌmpˌroup
leaf	nip	lif
mask	mæt	mæt
mouth	mau	mauf
music box	ˈmudɪˌbat	ˈmjuzɪkˌbat
nose	noud̥	nouz
squirrel	ʔu	fwuɪ
star	au	sʔaæ
string	ɪn	trɪŋ
sweater	ˈɛdu	fwɛtæ
television	ˈɛləˌbɪdə	ˈtɛləˌvɪʒən
that	dæʔ	dæt
thumb	ʌm	sʔʌm
toothbrush	ˈuˌbat	ˈtuˌbrʌʃ
truck	ʌ	trʌk
tub	ʌb̥	tʌb
vase	beɪt̟	veɪs
watch	wat	watʃ
yoyo	joujou	ˈjoujou
zipper	ˈdɪbu	ˈdɪpæ

* Tim's pre- and posttest responses have been reported in Hodson, Chin, Redmond and Simpson (in press), which presents a more in-depth case study of this child. Permission to reprint the list has been granted by the Journal of Speech and Hearing Disorders.

TIM

Basic Patterns	Pretest (5;0)	Posttest (6;1)
Syllable Reduction	5%	0%
Cluster Reduction	131	26
Prevocalic Singleton Obstruent Omission	42	5
Postvocalic Singleton Obstruent Omission	37	7
Stridency Deletion	100	18
Velar Deviation	100	17
/l/ Deviation	92	31
/r, ɚ/ Deviation	100	12
Nasal Deviation	5	0
Glide Deviation	50	0
Total	662	113
Average	66.2=66	11.3=11
Vowel Deviation	1 times	0 times
Prevocalic Voicing	6	0
Postvocalic Devoicing	4	1
Glottal Replacement	8	3
Backing	0	0
Stopping	19	5
Affrication	2	0
Deaffrication	3	1
Palatalization	0	0
Depalatalization	6	0
Coalescence	1	0
Epenthesis	1	0
Metathesis	0	0
Assimilation		
Nasal	0	0
Velar	0	0
Labial	3	3
Alveolar	0	0
"th"→/f, v, s, z/	0	3
Frontal Lisp	0	0
Dentalization of /t, d, n, l/	1	0
Lateralization	0	0
Other		
Nasal Addition/Replacement	6	0

ALAN: 5;11, 7;5

ALAN: 5;11, 7;5

Target	Pretest	Posttest
airplane	ˈwɛpwi	ˈɛupeɪn
basket	ˈbæwɛ	ˈbæskɪk
bed	bʌ	bɛd
candle	ˈnæwo	ˈkando
chair	tɛ	stjɛu
cowboy hat	ˈtaubɔɪwæ	ˈkaubɔɪˌhæt
crayons	na	ˈkwaænts
three	ti	twi
black	bæ	blæk
green	ɾi	gwɪn
yellow	ˈɛlou	ˈɛlou
doll	dau	dɑː

Target	Pretest	Posttest
page	peɪ	peɪts
quarter	ˈtɔuwə	ˈkwɔutə
rouge	wu	wuz
rug	wʌ	wʌg
Santa Claus	ˈtæwiˌta	ˈsæntəˌkɔz
skrewdriver	ˈtuˌdaɪwu	ˈskuˌdaɪvu
shoe	tu	sju
sled	pwɛ	swɛd
smooth	mu	smud
snake	ɹeɪ	sneɪk
soap	bou	soup
spoon	pʌn	spʌn

word		
feather	'bɛwə	'fɛdu
fish	tɪ	fɪʃ
flower	'bauwu	'fauwu
fork	bʌ	fouk
glasses	'dæwɛ	'glasɪz
glove	bʌ	gwʌv
gun	ʌ	gʌn
hanger	'eɪwu	'heɪɡu
horse	ʌ̃	hɔæs
ice cubes	'aɪtʃu	'aɪskʌbz
jumprope	'dɪ,ʔou	'dʒʌmp,woup
leaf	i	lif
mask	mæ	mæsk
mouth	ʌau	mauf
music box	'mu,ba	'muzɪk,baks
nose	mou	ɳouz̥

word		
spring	pɪ	spɪŋ
squirrel	tuwʌ	skwu:
star	tʌ̣	staæ
string	ɳɪ	swɪŋ
sweater	'pswu	'swɛtʊ̣
television	'bɛə,tɪjə	'tɛvə,vɪʒən
that	dæ	dæt
thumb	ʌ̃m	tʌm
toothbrush	'tu,bʌ	'tuf,bwaʃ
truck	tʌ̣	trʌk
tub	tʌ̣bʌ	tʌb
vase	beɪ	veɪs
watch	wa	wats
yoyo	'oɪwou	'ʌjʌ
zipper	'dɪpu	'zɪpʊ

ALAN

Basic Patterns	Pretest (5;11)	Postest (7;5)
Syllable Reduction	10%	0%
Cluster Reduction	106	26
Prevocalic Singleton Obstruent Omission	8	0
Postvocalic Singleton Obstruent Omission	97	0
Stridency Deletion	100	0
Velar Deviation	100	0
/l/ Deviation	92	69
/r, ɚ/ Deviation	100	88
Nasal Deviation	53	0
Glide Deviation	60	40
Total	736	223
Average	73.6=74	22.3=22
Vowel Deviation	5 times	4 times
Prevocalic Voicing	14	2
Postvocalic Devoicing	0	3
Glottal Replacement	1	0
Backing	0	0
Stopping	14	5
Affrication	0	1
Deaffrication	2	1
Palatalization	0	0
Depalatalization	4	3
Coalescence	0	0
Epenthesis	2	1
Metathesis	1	0
Assimilation		
Nasal ⁻	6	0
Velar	0	1
Labial	5	1
Alveolar	0	0
"th"→/f, v, s, z/	0	0
Frontal Lisp	0	0
Dentalization of /t, d, n, l/	0	0
Lateralization	0	0
Other		
Glide Syllable	13	0

BOBBY: 3;6, 4;5, 4;11

BOBBY: 3;6, 4;5, 4;11

Target	Pretest	Posttest	Re-eval.
airplane	ɑ	'ɛupwein	'ɛuplein
basket	ɑ	'bæksɪt+	'bæskɪt
bed	ɛ	bɛd	bɛd
candle	'uwə	'kændo	'kændo
chair	ɛ	tʃɛu	tʃɛu
cowboy hat	uɑ	'kaubɔɪˌhæt	'kaubɔɪˌhæt
crayons	o	'kweɪənz o+	'kweɪənz o̊
three	ɪ	fwi	θwi
black	ɑ	blæk	blæk
green	i	gwin	gwin
yellow	wʌ	'jɛwou	'jɛlou
doll	ɑ	dao	dɔlə
feather	u	'fɛðə	'fɛðə

Target	Pretest	Posttest	Re-eval.
page	u	peɪdʒ	peɪdʒ
quarter	'uwə	'kwoutu+	'kwɔutə
rouge	u	wuʒə	wuʒ
rug	ʌ	wʌg	wʌg
Santa Claus	'ɑˌwa	'sænti,kɔz+	'sæntəˌklɔz
skrewdriver	u,wa	'skwudwaɪvu+	'skwuˌdwaɪvu
shoe	u	ʃuə	ʃu
sled	ɛ	slɛd+	slɛd
smooth	u	smuð+	smuð
snake	eɪ	sneɪk+	sneɪk
soap	ou	ʃoup	soup
spoon	u	spun+	spun
spring	ɪ	spwiŋ+	spwiŋ

fish	ı	fıʃ	'fıʃ
flower	wa	'faʊwu	'flaʊwu
fork	ʊ	foʊk	foʊk
glasses	wa	gəˈlæsɪz	'glæsɪz
glove	ʌ	gəˈlʌv	glʌv
gun	ʌ	gʌn	gʌnə
hanger	jɛ	'hæŋə	'hæju
horse	ʌ	hoʊs	hoʊs
ice cubes	'aʊu	'aɪskjubz	'aɪskjubz
jumprope	'ʌ,ʌ	'dʒʌmpˌwoʊp	'dʒʌmpˌwoʊp
leaf	i	lif	lif
mask	æ	mæsk	mæsk
mouth	a	maʊθ	maʊs
music box	'u,a	'muvɪtˌbatʃ	'mjuzɪkˌbaks
nose	'noʊwə	noʊz	noʊz

squirrel	ʊ	skwɔə	skwʊʊ
star	a	'taʊwi	staʊ
string	ı	stwıŋ	stwıŋ
sweater	'ɛwə	'swɛtə	'swɛtu
television	'ʌ,u	'tɛləvıʒən	'tɛləˌvıʒən
that	a	ðæt	zæt
thumb	ʌm	θʌm	sʌm
toothbrush	'u,ʌ	'tuθˌbʌʃ	'tuθˌbwaʃ
truck	ʌ	twʌk	twʌk
tub	ʌ	tʌb	tʌb
vase	ʊ	veıs	veıs
watch	ja	watʃ	watʃ
yoyo	'oʊwoʊ	'joʊjoʊ	'joʊjoʊ
zipper	'ı,wu	'zıpu	'zıpu

BOBBY

Basic Patterns	Pretest (3;6)	Posttest (4;5)	Reevaluation* (4;11)
Syllable Reduction	71%	5%	0%
Cluster Reduction	171	14	0
Prevocalic Singleton Obstruent Omission	89	0	0
Postvocalic Singleton Obstruent Omission	100	0	0
Stridency Deletion	100	2	0
Velar Deviation	100	4	0
/l/ Deviation	100	54	15
/r, ɝ/ Deviation	100	100	96
Nasal Deviation	89	0	0
Glide Deviation	50	10	0
Total	970	189	111
Average	97	18.9=19	11
Vowel Deviation	14 times	0 times	0 times
Prevocalic Voicing	0	0	0
Postvocalic Devoicing	0	0	0
Glottal Replacement	0	0	0
Backing	0	0	0
Stopping	0	0	0
Affrication	0	0	0
Deaffrication	0	0	0
Palatalization	0	2	0
Depalatalization	0	0	0
Coalescence	0	0	0
Epenthesis	0	5	2
Metathesis	0	1	0
Assimilation			
Nasal	0	0	0
Velar	0	0	0
Labial	0	1	0
Alveolar	0	1	0
"th"→ /f, v, s, z/	0	1	3
Frontal Lisp	0	22	0
Dentalization of /t, d, n, l/	0	0	0
Lateralization	0	0	0
Other	0	0	0

*Bobby was available for re-evaluation six months
after his dismissal from the Phonology Program.

BARRY: 8;9, 8;10

BARRY: 8;9, 8;10

Target	Pretest	Posttest	Target	Pretest	Posttest
airplane	'ɛupʌn	'ɛʒpʌn	page	peɪtʃ	peɪdʒ
basket	'bɑkɪt	'bækɪt	quarter	'kɑtʊ	'kʌtə̬
bed	bɛd	bɛd	rouge	wutʃ	ruts
candle	'kænʊ	'kænd!	rug	wʌg̊	wʌg
chair	ʃɛu	ʃɛu	Santa Claus	tʃænɪˌkɔʃ	'sæntiˌkɔz
cowboy hat	'kaubɔɪˌhæt	'kaubɔɪˌhæt	skrewdriver	'ʃuˌdaɪdu	'suˌdavu
crayons	'kwɛɪənts	'kɹeɪənz̥	shoe	ʃu	ʃu
three	θwi	θwi	sled	sɛd	slɛd
black	blæk	blæk	smooth	muv	smuv
green	gwin	gwin	snake	tʃeɪk	tˢneɪk
yellow	'nɛdou	'ɛlou	soap	tʃoup	soup
doll	dɑː	dɑl	spoon	fʌn	spʌn

word		
feather	'fɛðu	'fɛðɚ
fish	fitʃ	fiʃ
flower	'faðu	'fawu
fork	fak	fouk
glasses	'gwæits	'gwæits
glove	gwʌb	glʌv
gun	gʌn	gʌn
hanger	'hæŋu	'hæŋu
horse	houts	houts
ice cubes	'aıkubts	'aıkubz
jumprope	'ʃʌmpıwoup	'zʌmpıwoup
leaf	lif	lif
mask	mæts	mæks
mouth	mauθ	mauθ
music box	'mudıˌbat	'mudıkˌbaks
nose	nouz	nouz
spring	fwiŋ	spriŋ
squirrel	tʃuu	ʃu:
star	tʃa	stau
string	tʃıŋ	'sriŋ
sweater	'sɛtu	'sɛtu
television	'tɛlaˌvinɛn	'tɛlaˌvinɛn
that	ðæt	ðæt
thumb	fʌm	fʌm
toothbrush	'tuˌbʌ	'tuˌbʌθ
truck	twʌk	twʌk
tub	tʌb	tʌb
vase	vʌts	vʌts
watch	watʃ	watʃ
yoyo	'ouou	'ʌlou
zipper	'wipu	'zipu

BARRY

Basic Patterns	Pretest (8;9)	Posttest (8;10)
Syllable Reduction	0%	0%
Cluster Reduction	66	43
Prevocalic Singleton Obstruent Omission	8	3
Postvocalic Singleton Obstruent Omission	13	7
Stridency Deletion	25	14
Velar Deviation	21	8
/l/ Deviation	77	38
/r, ɝ/ Deviation	100	77
Nasal Deviation	5	0
Glide Deviation	90	80
Total	405	290
Average	40.5=41	29
Vowel Deviation	4 times	1 times
Prevocalic Voicing	2	1
Postvocalic Devoicing	5	4
Glottal Replacement	0	0
Backing	0	0
Stopping	4	1
Affrication	14	7
Deaffrication	2	2
Palatalization	10	0
Depalatalization	1	4
Coalescence	6	1
Epenthesis	0	0
Metathesis	1	1
Assimilation		
Nasal	1	1
Velar	0	0
Labial	3	0
Alveolar	1	0
"th" → /f, v, s, z/	2	2
Frontal Lisp	0	0
Dentalization of /t, d, n, l/	0	0
Lateralization	0	0
Other	0	0

APPENDIX D

Sample Words for
Auditory Bombardment Lists

Final Consonants		Velars		Stridency and Final Consonant Clusters		
/p/	/t/	Final /k/ (& Final C)	Initial /k/	/ps/	/ts/	/ks/
mop	hat	book	cow	mops	hats	books
rope	bat	bike	car	ropes	bats	bikes
map	boat	lock	core	maps	boats	cokes
top	coat	rock	keg	tops	coats	cakes
cap	cat	coke	coke	caps	cats	rocks
tip	dot	cake	cake	tips	dots	rakes
pipe	gate	rake	cob	pipes	gates	tacks
lip	goat	rack	cook	lips	goats	locks
cup	mat	sack	come	cups	mats	sacks
type	note	tack	kiss	types	notes	racks

Stridency and Initial Consonant Clusters / Prevocalic Liquids

/sp/	/st/	/sm/	/sn/	/sk/	/l/	/r/
spot	store	smoke	snow	school	lock	rock
spout	stick	smile	snail	sky	log	rug
spur	stop	smell	snake	ski	luck	rack
spoon	stand	smear	sneeze	score	lake	rake
spy	stem	smog	snap	scope	leg	rook
speck	stork	smack	snack	skin	light	rye
space	steam	smudge	snob	skull	lip	rag
spark	star	smash	snag	scar	line	roll
spike	stamp	smooth	sneak	scale	lot	run
spook	stair	small	sniff	scarf	like	rain

* Ten words are given for each of the most commonly targeted phonological patterns. The child is to *listen* attentively (preferably with slight amplification) to approximately 15 words at the beginning and at the end of *each* session. The child must *not* repeat these words. (However, some words may overlap with the production practice list.) It is important to remember that individual children will have different needs (e.g., not every child will need to target final consonants or velars).

APPENDIX E

Suggested Experiential-Play
Activities for
Production Practice

The following activities make use of 5" x 8" picture cards drawn by the child depicting the words in which his current target phoneme or sequences will be produced.*

1. **Road.** Child lines cards up to make a road and drives a truck over the cards saying each words as he drives over it.

2. **Bean Bag.** Place cards on floor; child throws bean bag on cards and names the card he hit. He can also tell you which card he will try to hit before throwing the bean bag.

3. **Feed Clown.** Child says words to clown (large cardboard clown face with large hole for mouth) and then puts the cards in the clown's mouth. May be adapted to feeding cookies (cards) to Cookie Monster puppet.

4. **Fish.** Place paper clips on cards. Attach magnet on end of string attached to pole (cardboard, hanger, etc.). Child fishes for cards by touching paper clips with magnet. Child says word he will try to catch or has caught.

5. **Store.** Child buys his cards from the store clerk (you). Child tells you what he wants to buy.

6. **Hide 'n Seek.** Hide the cards in obvious places around the room. Child says words as he finds them.

7. **Bag of Cards.** Put all cards in a bag, child closes eyes and picks card out of bag and names it.

8. **Hook Game.** Bend the body of a coat hanger into a long, narrow pole-like form which you might wish to wind with colored yarn. Child puts rubber band around cards. This makes the cards bow. Child hooks rubber bands with the coat hanger hook and names cards. Good for final /k/ or front/back: "Hook the truck." "Pick up the truck with the hook." "The hook is stuck (on the rubber band)."

9. **Roll Ball.** Child rolls a ball on his cards and names the ones the ball rolled over.

10. **Bowling.** Stand up cards by leaning them against blocks. Child knocks down cards and names them.

11.   **Taking Pictures.** Child takes pictures of cards with camera (no film) and names them while doing so.

12.   **Flashlight.** Put cards in different places around room. Turn lights off. Child finds cards with flashlight and names them.

13.   **Mailbox.** Make mailbox. Child mails his cards while naming them.

14.   **Concentration.** Child and clinician both draw cards of same object. Place cards face down on table. Child and adult take turns trying to match the cards. Say cards while doing so.

15.   **What's Missing?** Put 2 or 3 cards on table. Child closes eyes. Adult takes one card away or turns one card over. Child guesses what card is missing.

16.   **Spinner Game.** Make a gameboard with the cards. Use anything as marker. Child spins spinner and moves the number of spaces, either saying each word as he moves, or saying the word he lands on.

17.   **Hopping.** Place cards on floor. Child hops from card to card, saying each one as he hops to it. (Hops next to, not on cards.)

18.   **TV Screen.** Make TV screen out of cardboard box, attach knob. Put cards in box. Child tells what card he sees on TV and can play with knobs (turn channel).

19.   **Sprinkle Speech Flowers.** Use sprinkling can. Put cards on floor. Child pretends they are flowers and *sp*rinkles the *sp*eech flowers. Especially good for /s/ clusters.

20.   **Card Games.** Make an "old maid" card. Child and adult hold cards in hand and pick from each other, guessing what they'll pick. You can also play a variety of card games that you make up yourself.

* This list was compiled by Therese Bednarz, Patricia Hall, Lynn Soprych-Krizic, Judy Sparks and Linda LaBuda Sustich, speech-language pathologists at South Metropolitan Association, Dolton, Il.

INDEX

This index cites the location of the major (A) Concepts and (B) Procedures discussed in this volume. Authors who are referenced are not indexed.

A: CONCEPTS